SEX THERAPY
HANDBOOK

SEX THERAPY HANDBOOK:
A Clinical Manual for the Diagnosis and Treatment of Sexual Disorders

Eric C. Krohne, Ph.D.

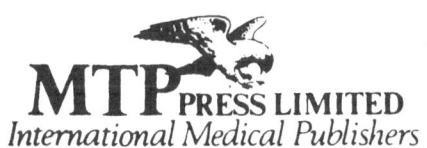

MTP PRESS LIMITED
International Medical Publishers

Published in the UK and Europe by
MTP Press Limited
Falcon House
Lancaster, England

Published in the US by
SPECTRUM PUBLICATIONS, INC.
175-20 Wexford Terrace
Jamaica, N.Y. 11432

ISBN 978-94-011-9666-6   ISBN 978-94-011-9664-2 (eBook)
DOI 10.1007/978-94-011-9664-2

Dedication

To my teachers

Richard Sewell & Gotthard Eberle

ERRATA SHEET

Note: Eight entries were left out of the Bibliography starting after Colgan, A. on page 91. They read as follows:

Connell, E. "Painful intercourse." Redbook, Dec. 1975, pp. 59-61.

Cooper, A. Some personality factors in frigidity. Journal of Psychosomatic Research, 1969, 13, 149-155.

Cornell medical index. Cornell University Medical College, New York: 1949.

Crist, T. Circumcision in the female. Journal of Sex Education and Therapy, 1977, 3 (1) 19-20).

Crist, T. Personal communication. 1980.

Croft, H.A. Causes of sexual dysfunction. Postgraduate Medicine, 1976, 60 (4), 193-198.

Croft, H.A. The sexual information examination. Journal of Sex and Marital Therapy, 1975, 1, 319-325.

DeMartino, M. Dominance--feeling, security--insecurity, and sexuality in women. In M. DeMartino, (Ed.), Sexual Behavior and Personality Characteristics. New York: Citadel Press, 1963.

Note: on page 92 of the Bibliography, the entries Fuchs, Furlow, Geboes, Goldberg, and Graber were erroneously repeated right after the Graber, B. entry.

Note: Figure 5 on page 59 and Figure 6 on page 72 were incorrectly placed in the book as turn pages. They should both be straight. All the above errors and miscellaneous spelling and punctuation errors which may appear in the text are the responsibility of the publisher.

ACKNOWLEDGEMENTS

I wish to express my appreciation to Peter Jager, Ph.D., who offered direction and encouragement while much of this material was being gathered for inclusion in my doctoral dissertation. I am also indebted to Doctors Masters and Johnson, and to their publisher, Little, Brown & Co., as well as to Farrar, Straus & Giroux, Inc., for allowing certain copywritten material to be reprinted in this text. Takey Crist, M.D., Walker Kirker, M.D., and Jeanne Kirker, R.N., M.N., generously provided me with previously unpublished clinical material, as did John Turner, M.A., who sketched the clinically descriptive illustrations. Connie Rhodes deserves particular acknowledgment for having typed, retyped, and re-retyped the manuscript—often working late into the evening and on weekends. Finally, I am grateful to Paul Williams, M.D., and Takey Crist, M.D., for their tutelage and friendship.

September 1, 1980
Jacksonville, N.C.

CONTENTS

SEX THERAPY
HANDBOOK

CHAPTER 1

An Historical Review of Sexual Pathology and Treatment

THE STORY OF ONAN

Some early sexual authorities viewed man's sexual behavior from a religio-philosophical framework which saw the physical and biological functions of the sex act as being secondary to the spiritual/moral issues involved. "Normal" sexual functioning was that which corresponded to certain religious or spiritual principles; "abnormal" or improper sexual functioning was that which diverted from these rules or traditions. Thus, we have the story of Onan (Genesis 38:8-10), who is reported to have ejaculated improperly, "spilling his seed on the ground" rather than impregnating his brother's widow as required by Jewish law. Interestingly, Onan's contemporaries interpreted his behavior as a voluntary contraceptive act -- either coitus interruptus or masturbation (Noonan, 1966). The Biblical narrative suggests that this improper and immoral sexual behavior angered the Hebrew god, who took Onan's life in retribution. (Onan certainly paid a high price for what might actually be one of the first recorded sexual dysfunctions -- premature ejaculation prior to vaginal penetration, an involuntary act.)

THE THIRTEENTH CENTURY

Later, the Western thinker Thomas Aquinas continued this moral tone in his sexual commentaries by refining the classical philosophical concept of Natural Law. On his terms, man's sexual behavior was proper so long as the goal was conception -- which he believed to be the natural outcome of coitus. However, because man's moral

1

Notes:

nature was seen as corrupt (concupiscent), his
sexual desires were often thought to be unnatural
and inappropriate -- especially when directed
toward recreation (fruitio) rather than procreation. Thus, for Thomas Aquinas, proper, normal,
and natural sexual functioning took place when
the sex act was intended for conception; all other
acts (i.e., those not intended solely for conception) were unacceptable due to their "unnatural"
self-indulgent character (Aquinas, 1947).

THE NINETEENTH CENTURY

By the eighteen hundreds some medical authorities were beginning to concern themselves with human sexual behavior. Like their predecessors, they
too believed that some sexual problems were just
functional, precipitated by such things as immod-
erate libidinal desires:

> Over-indulgence (sic) in intercourse...
> is sometimes the cause of barrenness;
> this is usually puzzling to the inter-
> ested parties, inasmuch as the prac-
> tices which, in their opinion, should
> be the source of numerous progeny,
> have the very opposite effect. By
> greatly moderating their ardor, this
> defect may be remedied. [Light and
> Life, p. 251].

Undoubtedly, this rather superficial perspective was due not only to the medical practitioners'
inadequate theoretical understanding of the subject but also to the primitive clinical procedures
of the period. For example, masturbation was seem
as a degenerative act, certain to end with the individual to complete physical and emotional col-
lapse. Note, in this regard, both the limited diagnostic rationale as well as the innocuous therapeutic suggestions contained in the following example:

> General Symptoms: The effects of
> ...self-pollution...appear in many forms
> ... In some cases, the only complaint
> the patient will make on consulting you
> is that he is suffering under a kind of
> continued fever. He will probably present
> a hot, dry skin with something of a hectic
> appearance. Though all the ordinary means
> of arresting such symptoms have been
> tried, he is one the better.
>
> The sleep seems to be irregular.

and unrefreshing -- restlessness during the
early part of the night and in the advanced
stages---profuse sweats before morning.
There is also frequent starting in the
sleep, from disturbing dreams. The characteristic feature is that your patient almost always dreams of sexual intercourse.
This is one of the earliest, as well as
most constant symptoms. When it occurs most
frequently, it is apt to be accompanied
with pain. A gleety discharge from the urethra may also be frequently discovered, especially if the patient is examined when at
stool or after urinating. Other common
symptoms are nervous headaches, giddiness,
ringing in the ears, and a dull pain in the
back of the head. It is frequently the case
that the patient suffers a stiffness in the
neck, darting pains in the forehead, and
also weak eyes are among the common symptoms.

Treatment: [The patient should be
instructed to]...sleep in a hard bed, and
rise early and take a sponge bath in cold
water every morning. Eat light suppers and
refrain from eating late in the evenings.
Empty the bladder thoroughly before retir-
ing, bathe the spine and hips with a sponge
dipped in cold water.

Never sleep lying on the back

Avoid all highly seasoned food and
read good books and keep the mind well employed. Take regular and vigorous outdoor
exercise every day.

Avoid all coffee, tea, wine, beer,
and all alcoholic liquors. Don't use to-
bacco, and keep the bowels free.

Prescription -- Ask your druggest to
put you up a good Iron Tonic and take it
regularly according to his directions.
[Light and Life, p. 457].

As medical science became more sophisticated,
so did physicians' understanding of sexual behavior and functioning. Unfortunately, the ac-
curacy of their understanding did not always improve proportionately to their increased sophis-
tication. The 1866 text, A Treatise on the Principles and Practices of Medicine, Diseases of
Women and Children and Medical Surgery, by W.
Paine, M.D. (Dean of the Faculty, the Philadelphia

Notes:

Notes:

University of Medicine and Surgery), is such a
case. However, these notations are of interest
because they illustrate not only the application
of the medical category of disease to what had
classically been considered moral problems, but
also because in them we see the advent of clinical
procedures, including chemotherapy and cauteriza-
tion, for the treatment of sexual problems. One
does wonder, though, about Paine's choice of sexual "pathologies" requiring treatment; and it is
interesting that he includes both functional (or
psychosexual) problems in the same chapter with
gonorrhea, balanitis, and syphilis -- perhaps indicating the possibility of a lingering moralism
behind the "clinical judgments" relating to spermatorrhoea, masturbation, nymphomania, and satyriasis.

Spermatorrhoea

By spermatorrhoea is understood
involuntary loss of semen. The most
frequent cause of this difficulty is
self-abuse; although it may be produced by everything that tends to ex-
cite the urino-genital organs; hence,
it may be induced by constipation,
ascaris in the rectum, hemorrhoids,
stricture of the urethra, excessive
venery, frequent use of mercurials,
and the habitual use of spirituous
liquors.

Symptoms: If spermatorrhoea be
associated with any considerable loss
of semen, it is followed by nervous
debility and irritability; constipation; dyspepsia; disturbed sleep;
despondency; hypochondria; epilepsy;
mental inertia; and insanity.

Treatment: There are but few
diseases where so much quackery has
been resorted to as in the management of this affection. Unprinci-
pled physicians are in the habit of
extorting large sums of money from
patients of this class under false
pretenses. The treatment consists in
removing the cause; hence, if produced by masturbation, the patient
should be informed of the fact, and
the practice prohibited. The bowels
should be regulated, and if parasites
infect the rectum, they should be
removed. The stomach should be kept
in a healthy condition, and frequent

baths and lively company enjoined. In
addition to the general bathing, the
genital organs should be showered in
cold water once or twice a day. The
specific remedies that have proved of
the greatest value in this disease,
are gelsemin, camphor, lupulin,
strychnin, viburin, ergot, canthoa-
rides, and phosphorous. These may be
caused either separately, or in such
combinations as the circumstances require. The topical applications consist in cauterizing the urethra by
means of Lallemand's porte caustique;
and the introduction of bougies, lub-
ricated with an ointment of hydrastin.
Quinine, iron, and general tonics also
have a favorable influence on this disease.

Masturbation

It can hardly be denied that there
are few habits that are more prevalent
or pernicious in their effects than masturbation. There is scarcely a practitioner of any considerable experience
and observation, who has not observed the
frequency in which it led to spermatorrhoea and nymphomania, with all their
terrible consequences. From the si-
lence which has been observed by medical writers and teachers relative to
these diseases, and the extensive practice of it at this period, we infer that
either the subject has been grossly neglected, or that masturbation is alarming-
ly on the increase. The practice of self-
pollution, when at first resorted to, has
but slight impression upon the constitution; but, if continued for a few
months, or years, at least, it produces
not only an abnormal condition of the
sexual organs, which results in nymphomania or spermatorrhoea, but affects
the nutritious functions, and lays the
foundation for scrofula, phthisis, and
insanity, besides so enfeebling the
general forces of the body as to predis-
pose the sufferer to many other mala-
dies.

Symptoms: The symptoms of masturbation are physical and intel-
lectual debility, irritable and va-
cillating dispositon, dyspepsia, constipation of the bowels, dry and husky

Notes:

Notes:

skin, scanty and high colored urine,
cold hands and feet, and an irregul-
ar and capricious appetite. If the
male abandons the practice in this
condition of the system, it will
soon be followed by involuntary
discharge of semen. At first this
will occur at night during lascivious dreams, but in time it will
occur during defecation and mictu-
rition. In this event there will be
atrophy of the testicles, cold and
shrivelled condition of the penis,
together with impotency. Or if the
impotency is not complete, the erec-
tions of the penis will be feeble,
and almost immediately followed by
emissions. In the female, where the
practice is abandoned, there will be
an irritability of the nervous system,
a tendency to irregularity of the
menses, leucorrhoea, prolapsus uteri,
and in many cases, frequent ovarian
excitement and discharge of the ovule.
If the disease be protracted, the
parts become weak, relaxed and cold,
and the patient averse to sexual intercourse.

Nymphomania

Nymphomania is a disease of females, consisting of an irresistible
desire for sexual intercourse. It
more frequently occurs in those of a
nervous, irritable habit; or of a
dark, scrofulous, or tuberculous constitution. It is produced by masturbation; the reading of lascivious
books; high, stimulating living; an
absence of physical and mental em-
ployment; parties, gay company;
uterine and vaginal irritation; hemorrhoids, and the presence of parasites in the rectum. In the major-
ity of cases, this condition is never
made manifest by the patient; but in
others, the feelings of modesty are
overcome, and she gives vent to the
most obscene expressions, and im-
modest and disgusting manifestations.
It may amount to absolute insanity, or
only an irritable and passionate condition of the mind; while in other
cases, the patient seeks to satiate
her morbid passion by sexual commerce,
or self-abuse. It soon, however,

Notes:

undermines the constitution, producing
an irritable condition of the bowels
and digestive organs, disorganization
of the blood, tuberculous degeneration,
haemoptysis, deranged menstrual functions, leucorrhoea, lumbago, constipation, melancholy, pulmonary consumption,
and death.

Treatment: The treatment consists
in removing the cause, invigorating
and toning the stomach and bowels, hot
sitz baths, cold vaginal injections,
and the cauterizing of the clitoris
with argenti nitras, in cases where
the disease has been produced by masturbation. Senecin and gelsemin, in
the proportion of two grains of the
former to one-tenth of a grain of the
latter, two or three times a day, exerts a specific influence over the
disease, and I have cured many bad
cases with it. Quinine, iron, and
crypipedin, also exert a favorable
impression.

Satyriasis

Satyriasis is an insatiable desire for sexual intercourse. This is
a species of nervous disease produced
by a disordered condition of the
cerebellum, caused by alcoholic
drinks, high living, excessive venery, and a large development of the
base of the brain. It can be cured
by a low diet, frequent shower baths,
physical out-door labor, ice-bags to
the cerebellum, a hard bed, and hop
pillows [Paine, 1866, pp. 919-
921].

THE TWENTIETH CENTURY

The Psychoanalysts

Apparently the general thrust of medicine's
sexual theories and clinical procedures continued in much these same ways for the next several
generations, leading one physician, Wilhelm
Reich, to say in March of 1919, "Perhaps it is
the moralism with which the subject is approached
that disturbs me" (Reich, 1975, p. 18). Later,
however, after psychoanalytic training, Reich
left the practice of general medicine for psychiatry and sex research:

Notes:

> One has to be familiar with this atmosphere in the fields of sexology and psychiatry before Freud to understand the enthusiasm and relief which I felt when I encountered him. Freud has paved a road to a clinical understanding of sexuality. He showed that adult sexuality proceeds from stages of sexual development in childhood. It was immediately clear: sexuality and procreation are not the same. The words "sexual" and "genital" could not be used interchangeably. The sexual experience comprises a far greater realm than the genital experience, otherwise perversion such as pleasure in coprophagy, in filth, or in sadism could not be called sexual. Freud exposed contradictions in thinking and brought in logic and order. [Reich, 1975, p. 25][1]

As Reich stated so clearly, with Freud sexual theory expanded to include every sphere of human activity. He developed new perspectives from which to view human sexuality (psychoanalytic theory), as well as techniques (psychoanalytic psychotherapy) for the clinical application of therapeutic principles. In his terms, man's sex drive was seen as a natural characteristic of human behavior, and sexual difficulties or abnormalities were identified as pathological, requiring treatment. In short, not only did Freud develop a comprehensive theory of libido, but he also precisely spelled out how psychoanalysts should observe and understand the behavior of the patient so they could guide their patients (usually through lengthy and expensive therapy) toward an appropriate adjustment.

The Behaviorists

Working from a quite different perspective, psychological researchers from the behavioral schools had, by the late nineteen-fifties and sixties, begun theoretical formulations and clinical experimentation in the area of human sexuality. They hypothesized that sexual dysfunctions were conditioned responses to anxiety-provoking sexual stimuli which could be treated by reversing or "deconditioning" the individual through systematic desensitization techniques (e.g., Wolpe, 1958, 1969; and Lazarus, 1963). The results of their

---

[1]Quoted with permission of Farrar, Straus & Giroux.

experiments were quite positive, often with better
than a 75% success rate in correcting psychogenic
sexual disorders (Seagraves, 1976); this was usually achieved in only a fraction of the time required by classical analysis.

The New Sex Therapists

Paralleling and systematizing the experimental developments of these behaviorists and others
(e.g., Robie, 1925, 1927; Kelly, 1930, 1953; and
Semans, 1956) was the clinical work of Masters
and Johnson (Human Sexual Response, 1966; Human
Sexual Inadequacy, 1970) whose pioneering achieve-
ments are virtually responsible for making sex
therapy into a contemporary health care specialty.
They viewed nonorganically based sexual dysfunctions as learned disorders precipitated (primarily) by sexual ignorance, performance anxiety,
and poor communication between partners. This
understanding caused them to develop short-term
treatment programs consisting of directive psychotherapy, communication training, sex education,
and a type of systematic (in vivo) desensitization through a series of sensate focus exercises
(Franks and Wilson, 1974).

Closely following the lead of Masters and
Johnson is the work of Hartman and Fithian
(Treatment of Sexual Dysfunction, 1972), who incorporate much of the former's methodology into
a "bio-psycho-social" diagnostic/treatment format. This approach uses psychological testing
to achieve a sexual diagnosis as well as the physical examinations so characteristic of Masters
and Johnson; it also structures treatment around
behavioral tasks and sex education, while de-emphasizing -- without totally discounting -- psychotherapy and/or relationship counseling. This
latter factor has led at least one prominent sex
therapist (Ellis, 1975) to suggest that while
Hartman and Fithian are "highly creative," their
treatment procedures are superficial (i.e., most-
ly "diversionary") and as clinicians, they are
prone to "risk-taking." Such criticism notwithstanding, many therapists who have been trained
by Hartman and Fithian continue to employ the
bio-psycho-social approach on a regular and (sup-
posedly) successful basis -- thus placing it a-
mong the major approaches in modern sex therapy.

In 1974 Helen Kaplan published The New Sex
Therapy wherein she described a therapeutic
schema which tied together the directive-behav-
ioral-educative orientations of Masters and
Johnson/Hartman and Fithian and the dynamic
theories of the psychoanalysts. From this

Notes:

Notes:

perspective sex therapy begins with the "new" ra-
pid treatment approaches; but clinical intervention may also occur at deeper levels (via intensive individual and/or conjoint psychotherapy) so
as to modify those intrapsychic or relational conflicts that may also be involved in the sexual disorder.

Here, then, beginning with the analytical theories of Freud and continuing on through the exper-
imentations of the behaviorists and the procedural
formulations of Masters and Johnson, to the new
pervasive psychotherapeutic approach of Helen
Kaplan, is seen the evolution of modern sex therapy. From a lengthy analytical treatment by singularly trained experts, sex therapy (which had been
only a sub-category) developed into a new cross-
disciplined specialty: the short-termed clinical
treatment of psychosexual dysfunction.

CHAPTER 2

The Human Factors in Sex Therapy

THE THERAPIST

Ideally, all clinicians practicing sex therapy will have had extensive training in counseling theories and procedures. This is advantageous because counseling skills are just as important in the treatment of psychosexual dysfunctions as they are when doing individual psychotherapy, conjoint marriage counseling, or any one of the various types of group therapy (cf. Sager, 1975). As a matter of fact, depending on the circumstances, sexual "counseling" or "therapy" (terms often used interchangeably) may require any or all of these counseling modalities, so the more experienced and capable clinicians are, the more likely it is that they will be able to respond adequately to the sexual problems that are presented in clinical practice.

Sexual comfort and discomfort

In addition to the usual skills required of most counselors, sex therapists must also be comfortable with sexual issues. Primarily this means that they must be comfortable with their own sexuality. If this most basic requirement cannot be met, it is doubtful that they will perform competently as sex therapists (cf. Reed, 1976). After all, how can counselors encourage masturbation, as has been the classical procedure with pre-orgasmic women, if they feel guilty about or are unable to masturbate themselves?

A common place for the clinician's discomfort with sexual material is to be seen in the area of vocabulary. Often patients describe their problems in the vernacular; the sexually

Notes:

anxious therapist typically feels the need to "correct" these terms, translating them into "acceptable" clinical (sterile) language. Unfortunately these "clinical translations" may make patients feel unclean, raise their anxiety, and make it even more difficult for them to disclose relevant material for fear of making another "dirty" comment. A less anxious therapist would attempt to use a vocabulary that is comfortable to the patients, questioning their choice of terms only when those words were too vague to be meaningful. (Such might be the case when a woman enters therapy complaining of breast pain during "lovemaking." In this context is unclear if she means that her breast(s) hurt during intercourse, during oral or manual nipple stimulation, or while doing any number of other intimate acts.)

Clearly, then, the therapist's comfort or discomfort with sexual issues will become evident in the clinical setting. When discomfort is the case, direct confrontation must be undertaken. Psychotherapy, either dynamic or behavioral, is often successful; the S.A.R. (Sexual Attitude Reassessment) seminars offered by various training centers throughout the country have also been helpful in this area (Chilgren and Briggs, 1973), but it is not yet clear if their effect is sufficiently long lasting.

If the clinician's sexual anxiety has not been satisfactorily resolved, it is likely that it will become the liability of the patient. For example, the anxious therapist might comment, "I know that some people engage in oral-genital contact, but I disapprove; in fact, it has been my experience that only homosexuals, or people with latent homosexual tendencies, do that kind of thing." Obviously such a statement is communicating the speaker's own discomfort with oral-genital contact and/or homosexuality, or both. And, because the listener most probably believes that the therapist is an authority on "what is sexually normal," great psychological pain, anxiety and guilt may be the result.

THE DYSFUNCTIONAL PATIENTS

There is an infinite variety of sexual problems. However, all psychosexual dysfunctions share in common the same cause: **anxiety**. This is the case even though common sense and personality theories tell us that the origins and manifestations of the particular symptoms are most probably unique with each patient and/or within each sexual relationship.

The focus of therapy.

Depending on the circumstances, therapy may focus either on the dysfunctional individual or on the sexual relationship wherein the problem occurs. Sex therapy regularly focuses on the dysfunctional individual in cases of personal anxiety, such as with many preorgasmic women (cf. Barbach, 1975). With other types of sexual problems, where the dysfunction is believed to stem from the patient's sexual relationship (secondary orgasmic dysfunction, dyspareunia or vaginismus of sudden onset, etc.), the therapeutic focus is on the couple's interaction -- and both persons should enter therapy on a joint basis.

In cases where the dysfunction is a reaction to problems or attitudes within the relationship, the inadequacy is approached by treating the relationship through techniques not unlike those classically used in marital therapy. In other circumstances, sexual dysfunctions may be symptoms of chronic sexual anxieties that only present themselves within the relationship, having their origins elsewhere (in childhood, sexual ignorance, etc.). These anxieties are often treated successfully with simple sex education. When this is not sufficient, the dysfunctional patient may require individual psychotherapy in addition to the couple's relationship counseling and the joint performance of prescribed behavioral tasks.

In short, some sexual problems can be treated on an individual basis. However, because sexual dysfunctions usually surface within a relationship, it is often necessary to treat the couple rather than just the individual presenting the dysfunctional symptoms. Variations on the focus of sex therapy will be made later in this text.

THE THERAPIST/PATIENT RELATIONSHIP

In treating psychosexual dysfunction, the therapeutic task requires that the therapist and the sexually anxious patient(s) develop a relationship that will allow for and encourage enough self-disclosure so that the patient(s) can work toward identifying and resolving the anxiety that is precipitating the sexual problem. This type of interchange is not just "clinical interaction" between individuals, but rather it is to be a genuine sharing between patient(s) and advocate/mediator (the therapist) within a relationship based on support and acceptance.

Notes:

The clinical therapeutic relationship

Naturally, a formal clinical relationship (with all of its professional and legal dimensions) begins by virtue of the fact that the therapist and the patients have started working together in a clinical setting. However, a genuinely therapeutic relationship (wherein healing occurs) begins only after a mutual bond of trust and respect has developed that will support the patients in the risking of self-disclosure that precedes all authentic behavioral change. Hopefully, this bond will be established early in the relationship; ideally, it will start during the taking of the history so that the clinician will have an accurate view of the patient's sexual development and intimate relationships. Should the therapeutic relationship not be established this early, the history, or part of it, may need to be retaken.

CHAPTER 3

The Psychophysiology of Human Sexual Response

SEXUAL PSYCHOPHYSIOLOGY

Theory

The "new" or directive sex therapies, as characterized by the writings of Masters and Johnson (1966, 1970), Hartman and Fithian (1972), and Helen Kaplan (1974b), incorporate elements of the psychodynamic therapies (the use of insight, individual and relationship counseling, etc.) and behaviorism (especially desensitization, conditioning techniques, and educational procedures) with their own research findings and treatment perspectives to formulate strategies for the short-term treatment of psychosexual dysfunction. The basis for this new approach has been Masters and Johnson's classic laboratory studies in the area of human sexual response. Their findings (1966) contributed the essential phenomenological description of human sexual psychophysiology that serves even today as the foundation for the clinical understanding of sexual function and dysfunction.

Research

The first scientifically reliable studies of human sexual behavior were conducted under the direction of A. Kinsey (1947, 1948 and 1953), but these were limited to a sociological perspective and derived totally from interrogation. Masters and Johnson, on the other hand, undertook psychophysiological studies that sought to describe the pattern of human sexual response on the basis of direct observation and recorded physiologic variables. Their 1966 text pictures both the male and female sexual responses as intensifying reactions to sexual stimuli which they arbitrarily divided into four specific phases: 1) excitement,

15

Notes:

2) plateau, 3) orgasm, and 4) resolution (Figs. 1 and 2 p. 17). This division provided Masters and Johnson with an effective framework wherein they could thoroughly detail the variations and changes in the sexual response cycle (1966, p. 4).

Human Sexual Response: Classical Description

Excitement phase

Either erotic fantasy or tactile stimulation can produce penile erection in the human male. When this happens there is a lengthening of the urethra, both testes elevate within the scrotal sac, and there is considerable tensing and thickening of the scrotal integument.

Females usually evidence a mucoid transudate (a lubricating fluid) in the vagina within thirty seconds of satisfactory somatic or psychic stimulation. This sexual tension brings on a vascular engorgement that produces a swelling in both the glans and the shaft of the clitoris. Nipple erection and enlargement, and an increase in breast size also result from this stimulation. In and around the outer vagina, the labia minora swell and the labia majora tend to flatten. Inwardly, the vaginal barrel extends and expands.

Plateau phase

If effective sexual excitement continues, the diameter of the male's corona glans (the "head" of the penis) increases somewhat, and the testes swell and continue to elevate. Some fluid from the Cowper's gland may also be emitted from the penis at this time.

In the female, the vaginal engorgement which began during the excitement phase continues during plateau. This brings on a shrinkage of the outer third of the lumen which allows the vagina to actually "grip" even a very small penis during penetration. The uterus moves upward within the pelvic area as the vagina expands with continued vasocongestion. The previously elongated clitoris then begins to shrink and retreat from the vaginal opening, and the labia minora undergo a noticeable "reddening." At this point orgasm is impending if adequate stimulation continues.

Orgasmic phase

Males usually become aware that orgasm is imminent as they feel the ejaculate collect in the prostatic urethra; however, the orgasm actually begins only when the periurethral musculature

Male and Female Sexual Response Cycles[1]   Notes:

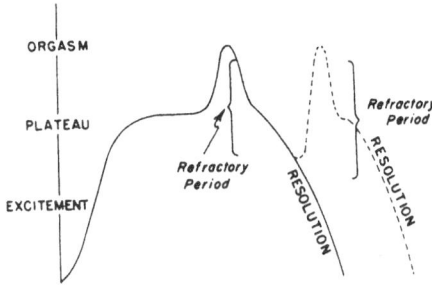

Figure 1:   The male sexual response cycle.

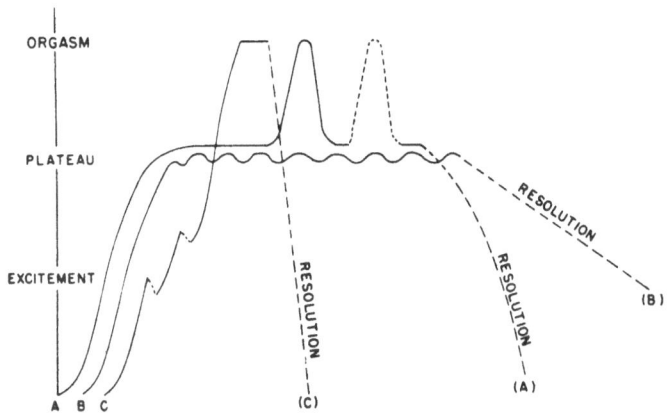

Figure 2:   The female sexual response cycle.

---

1. Since the male sexual response varies only in
    duration, a single pattern (Fig. 1) is de-
    scriptive of their response cycle. Females,
    on the other hand, vary in both intensity and
    duration; therefore, three simplified patterns
    (Fig. 2) are used to describe their typical
    response. The sexual response cycles shown
    above are taken from Masters and Johnson
    (1966, p. 5), and are used with their permis-
    sion, and with permission of their publisher,
    Little, Brown & Co.

Notes:

undergoes a series of involuntary contractions.
Similarly, ejaculation results from a series of
rhythmic contractions of the urethral bulb and the
penile urethra.

During orgasm the female undergoes a series
of contractions involving the muscles of the outer
third of the vagina. Deeper within the pelvis,
the uterus also contracts rhythmically.

Both men and women note that orgasm causes
an increase in pulse, respiration and blood pressure.
The "sex flush" (the reddening reported during
plateau) also spreads and becomes more intense
during this experience.

Resolution phase

Following orgasm the male quickly loses his
erection. This happens in two stages: in the
first stage penile size decreases rapidly but in-
completely; in the second stage the penis returns
slowly to its normal size. The testes and scrotum
then drop to their original position; pulse, blood
pressure, and respiration soon return to normal;
the sex flush quickly disappears.

After orgasm the man goes through a refrac-
tory period wherein he is unable to become restimulated. This period varies in duration from person
to person -- usually taking longer as the individual ages.

Within half an hour after her orgasm the woman's areolae, clitoris, uterus, and vaginal barrel
shrink to their original size. Unlike the male,
however, the female does not experience refraction,
and she is capable of another orgasm almost immediately.

SEXUAL RESPONSE PATTERN: THEORETICAL ALTERNATIVES

Biphasic Sexual Response

Helen Kaplan has repeatedly (1974a, 1974b,
1975 and 1976) pointed out her belief that Masters
and Johnson's quadriphasic model wrongly implies
that the human sexual response is an orderly sequence of a unitary and inseparable event. Initially (1974a, 1974b, and 1975) she was of the o-
pinion that a biphasic pattern -- unlike that of
Masters and Johnson in that it included the entire
sexual response cycle(s) in just the excitement
and orgasm phases -- more accurately described sexual psychophysiology (Fig. 3, p. 19: "Sexual response is...actually a well coordinated sequence
of two discreet physiologic responses: erection

Human Sexual Response: Kaplan's View[1]   Notes:

Figure 3: Biphasic sexual response (male and female).

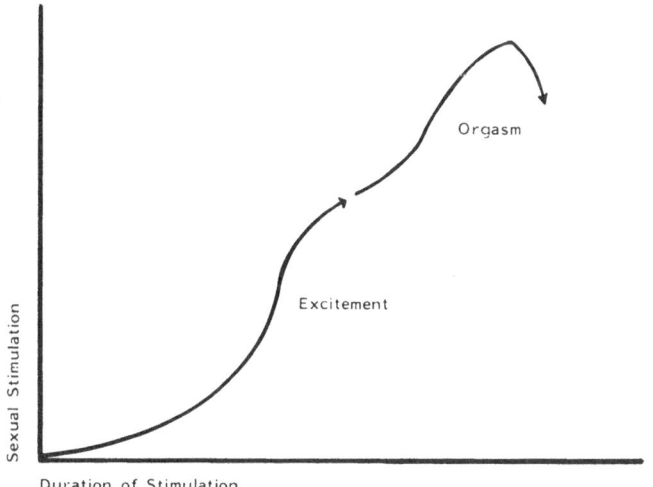

Figure 4: Triphasic sexual response (male and female).

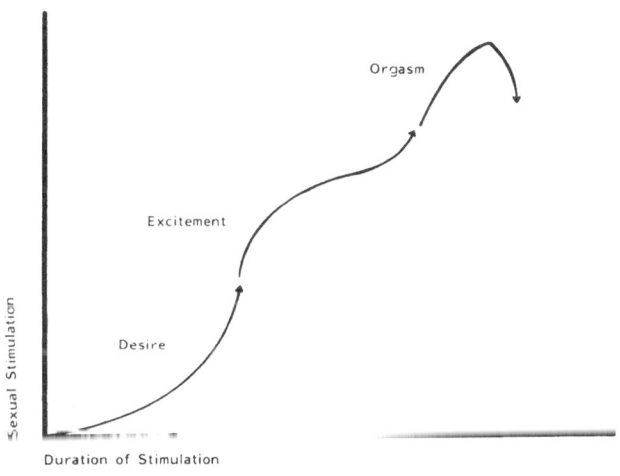

1. Figures 3 and 4 illustrate Kaplan's contention
    that the sexual response cycle is a sequence
    of discreet psychophysiologic responses.

Notes:

and ejaculation in the male, and analogously,
lubrication-swelling and orgasm in the female"
(1974a, p. 126).

Triphasic Sexual Response

Later (1976, 1977 and 1979) Kaplan expanded
her view to include a (pre-excitement) desire
phase. This final, triphasic scheme (Fig. 4, p.
19) was theoretically an improvement over both
the classical model of Masters and Johnson, and
her own earlier (biphasic) description, in that
it allowed for the incorporation of various sexual appetites (hyperlibido, hypolibido, etc.)
within the sphere of human sexual responses -- a
move she calls "entirely consistent with a psychophysiologic theoretical orientation" (1976,
p. 84). Unfortunately, however, in the absence
of either confirming psychophysiologic studies
or other supporting clinical evidence,[1] neither
Kaplan's biphasic nor triphasic descriptions of
the sexual response cycles have been shown to be
more accurate or more useful than that previously offered by Masters and Johnson, and neither
has become widely accepted in sex therapy cir-
cles.

---

[1]Kaplan admits (1977) that her psychophysiologic descriptions of the male/female sexual response cycles are unsupported in studies on hu-
mans, and her final triphasic construct is simply a "hypothesis...based on fragments of clinical evidence and animal experiments and by analo-
gy with the physiology of other human appetites"
(p. 4).

CHAPTER 4

Sexual Function and Dysfunction

ADEQUATE AND INADEQUATE SEXUAL FUNCTIONING

Sexual Adequacy

Researchers and therapists have been unable to clinically determine or universally agree upon what constitutes normal or adequate sexual functioning. Lazarus (1969, p. 53), however, offers a definition of sexual adequacy that is applicable to and operable within most theoretical and/or clinical perspectives. In his terms, sexual adequacy is "the ability to obtain and maintain a sufficient degree of sexual arousal so as to derive pleasure from the sex act and contribute to the enjoyment of one's partner, finally leading to orgasmic release."[1] (This suggests that an adequate sexual response closely resembles the psychophysiologic response pattern described by Masters and Johnson.) Interestingly, Lazarus does not state the types of behavior, or describe the techniques by which this pleasure is to be achieved, leading one to infer that the way sexual pleasure is obtained is to be determined by the needs and desires of the individuals concerned.

---

[1]Lazarus' requirement of orgasmic release is the only controversial element in his definition. Most therapists recognize that orgasmic response is not necessarily a personal goal of every person, in every sexual relationship, all the time. Therefore, on occasion, one may choose to modify this part of the definition if it is not applicable to the needs or goals of the patient(s) involved.

Notes:

Sexual Inadequacy

A sexual response that fails to meet the expectations of either partner is often -- though
not always accurately -- termed "inadequate." Occasionally the sexual response of any person can
be variously impaired, affecting both performance
and one's subjective evaluation of those experiences. When such an impairment actually interrupts
or significantly changes an individual's normal
sexual response cycle, it is termed a sexual dysfunction.[1] At other times, however, the supposed
"inadequacy" is simply the result of unrealistic
expectations that cannot be fulfilled. In these
cases the problem lies with the inappropriate expectations, rather than with the psychophysiology
of the sexual response cycle.

IDENTIFICATION/CLASSIFICATION OF SEXUAL DYSFUNCTIONS

Unfortunately there is no universally accepted method or rationale for the clinical identifica-
tion of human sexual disorders, and although various
systems of classification have been recommended
(Croft, 1976; Kaplan 1974a; and O'Connor, 1976;
etc.), none has been broadly applied in the professional literature, and no single formulation
has come into general clinical use. In fact, a
thorough review of the sex therapy literature reveals that sexual dysfunctions are most often identified simply by the psychophysiologic symptoms
they exhibit (Hartman and Fithian, 1972: Masters
and Johnson, 1970; Meyer, 1976; Zussman and Zussman,
1976; etc.) and then they are often grouped according to the gender of the patients wherein they occur -- when that designation is essential to, or
characteristic of, the disorder.

---

[1]Sexual dysfunction can be termed either
primary (when the impairment has always existed)
or secondary (when it occurs after a period of
sexual adequacy). Situationally precipitated im-
pairments are considered secondary dysfunctions
since they follow a period of adequate sexual
functioning.

PSYCHOSEXUAL DYSFUNCTIONS: MALE   Notes:

Impotence

A male is considered sexually impotent when he cannot obtain or maintain an erection of the penis suitable for vaginal penetration[1] and pleasurable coitus (Meyer, 1976).

Primary impotence

Males who have <u>never</u> experienced satisfactory coitus, with orgasm, are conisdered to be suffering from primary impotence. This is the case even though they may relate a history of satisfactory masturbation to orgasm. The American Medical Association (1972) notes that primary impotence is usually not precipitated by any single factor, but rather, it is often attributable to a cluster of influences such as family environment, peer relationships, negative maternal influences, religious beliefs, homosexual contacts, and self-devaluation following negative experiences with prostitutes. Furthermore, if the first unsuccesful coital attempt is tied to trauma, an on-going pattern of failure may develop.

Secondary impotence

Erectile difficulties arising <u>after</u> a period of adequate sexual functioning comprise the category of secondary impotence. Anxiety is the most common etiological factor in this sexual dysfunction, even though drugs, alcohol, diabetes, and diffuse arteriosclerosis may be occasionally involved. O'Connor and Stern (1972) suggest that complaints of inconsistent or selective potency, partial or infirm erection, and/or reactive impotence (e.g., following a 14 point drop in the Dow Jones average) are all descriptive of secondary impotence.

Premature ejaculation

Two different criteria are frequently applied when distinguishing between "fast" or "quick" ejaculation and premature ejaculation. One factor used by many clinicians in establishing that an ejaculation is actually premature, is the <u>amount of time</u> required, after sexual

---

[1]Masters and Johnson (1970) make an interesting observation regarding penile penetration. On their terms it is not necessary that the penis successfully penetrate a vagina; rather, they suggest that any successful intromission, either heterosexual or homosexual, designates potency -- on

Notes:

stimulation begins, before the male ejaculation. O'Connor (1976) reports that an ejaculatory delay of 1-1/2 - 2 minutes, after vaginal penetration, cannot be considered premature. Some other clinicians feel, however, that the number of penile/vaginal thrusts that take place before ejaculation occurs is the distinguishing factor in premature ejaculation. O'Connor and Stern (1972) and O'Connor (1976) note that an ejaculatory delay of more than ten thrusts is not premature. Jon Meyer (1976), on the other hand, suggests that an ejaculation any time prior to, or during, the first fifteen thrusts is premature.[1]

Primary premature ejaculation

Fast ejaculatory responses are frequently a problem for young males who have not yet learned techniques for delaying their ejaculations. Most often, however, these "quickies" are not of dysfunctional proportions. This being the case, primary premature ejaculation is not a common problem.

Secondary premature ejaculation

Premature ejaculation is almost always a secondary development. That is to say, it is a sexually dysfunctional behavior that is precipitated by situational factors and reinforced by repetition.

---

[1]In Meyer's terms it is also a premature ejaculation when the ejaculation happens during foreplay (if both partners had intended to continue on to coitus) and/or when the ejaculation occurs during, or just before, vaginal penetration.

Retarded ejaculation

This psychophysiologic disorder, which was earlier termed "ejaculatory incompetence" by Masters and Johnson (1970), has been defined by Helen Kaplan (1974b, p. 316) as a "specific inhibition of the ejaculatory reflex." Jon Meyer (1976) portrays retarded ejaculation as a profoundly slow ejaculatory response during coitus which, in some males, is characterized by a complete inability to ejaculate intravaginally -- with the masturbatory response usually not affected.[1] J.F. O'Connor (1976) feels that this dysfunction is clinically established when a male cannot ejaculate within 45 minutes after vaginal penetration.

It was originally reported (Masters and Johnson, 1970) that retarded ejaculation was a very rare condition. This impression was later confirmed by O'Connor and Stern (1972) who reported that retarded ejaculation occurred only once in every 15,000 males. Since then, however, Kaplan (1974b) and O'Connor (1976) have re-examined this phenomenon and both have concluded that it is more prevalent than previously thought.

Primary and secondary retarded ejaculation

Masters and Johnson (1970) note that retarded ejaculation presents itself in both primary and secondary forms; and while Helen Kaplan agrees that, in its secondary form, this dysfunction is not uncommon, she suggests that primary retarded ejaculation is only rarely encountered in clinical practice. Thus, it seems safe to conclude that this sexual disorder is most often brought on by situational factors and maintained as a learned or conditioned response.

PSYCHOSEXUAL DYSFUNCTIONS: FEMALE

Orgastic Dysfunction

Perhaps the most widely recognized sexual disorder in women has been the inability to achieve orgasm. At one time this was referred to

---

[1]Helen Kaplan (1974b) notes that there are cases of more severe inhibition where the man cannot ejaculate in the presence of a woman -- even with masturbation. Even in these cases, however, the masturbatory ejaculation is usually not affected if he is allowed complete isolation from females.

Notes:

as "frigidity," but the pejorative nature of that term (which was supposed to designate only an inhibition of the orgastic component of the female sexual response cycle) has led to its being replaced in the clinical nomenclature. "Orgastic dysfunction" or "non-orgasmia" are the terms most often applied.

Primary orgastic dysfunction: Preorgasmia

Women who have never experienced orgasm by any means (masturbation, cunnilingus, coitus, etc.) evidence primary orgastic dysfunction. Because all healthy women with normal anatomy are -- theoretically -- potentially able to experience orgasm, those with primary symptoms might more accurately be termed "preorgasmic" since their initial orgasmic response still awaits them.

Secondary orgastic dysfunction

If orgastic dysfunction occurs after a period of orgasmic response, it is considered a secondary disorder. As Kaplan (1974b) has pointed out, secondary orgastic dysfunctions may be either absolute or situational. When the woman cannot achieve orgasm under any circumstances, the disorder is absolute; if she cannot reach climax on some occasions, but she can on others, it is a situational orgastic dysfunction.

Dyspareunia

Painful coitus may be either organic or psychological in origin, and it may present itself as either a primary or secondary dysfunction.

Rubin (1968) reports that about one-fifth of all the women who have been treated surgically for prolapse of the uterus experience a loss of feeling or pain during coitus as a result of those procedures. Jeffcoate (1967) notes a 30% incidence of apareunia and dyspareunia subsequent to combined anterior and posterior colporrhaphy. Masters and Johnson (1970) have found that vulvovaginitis, endometriosis, and pelvic infections can also bring on painful intercourse.

Primary dyspareunia

As a primary disorder dyspareunia may originate as an anxiety reaction to a woman's first experience of intercourse. Other causes, such as an intact hymen, may cause pain during her first sexual experience, and the anticipation of more pain on subsequent occasions may keep her from adequate sexual functioning thereafter.

Secondary dyspareunia

Emotions or physical trauma may precipitate secondary dyspareunia. For example, a woman's occasional anger toward her sexual partner may interrupt her normal sexual response cycle, causing inadequate vaginal lubrication, resulting in painful intercourse. Episiotomy scars and changes in the size of the vagina following hysterectomy are also common causes of secondary dyspareunia.

Vaginismus

An involuntary spasm of the perivaginal musculature (specifically, the sphincter vaginae and levator ani muscles), which happens whenever an attempt at vaginal penetration is made, is termed vaginismus. This reflex (conditioned response) of the muscles surrounding the vaginal opening makes penetration very difficult or virtually impossible.

On those occasions when vaginal penetration is accomplished, the woman experiences little, if any, sexual excitement (O'Connor, 1976) and the resulting coital activities are not pleasurable for her. As with orgastic dysfunction, however, she must not be automatically designated "frigid." Indeed, Kaplan (1974b) correctly points out that "many women who seek treatment for vaginismus are sexually responsive. They may be orgastic on clitoral stimulation, enjoy sexual play, and seek sexual contact -- as long as this does not lead to intercourse" (p. 412 - 413).

Primary vaginismus

This involuntary muscular response is not limited to sexual activity; when the precipitating anxiety is present, vaginismic symptoms will present themselves whenever vaginal penetration is attempted. This means that some women have never been able to undergo a pelvic examination or use a tampon because this disorder sometimes surfaces early in life.

Secondary vaginismus

Relational problems, sexual anxiety, severe dyspareunia, and/or sexual trauma, etc., can bring on secondary vaginismus. Fortunately, however, both primary and secondary vaginismus are rare disorders (Kaplan, 1974b) and some sex therapists have never been called upon to treat them.

Notes:

General sexual dysfunction

A female who is essentially devoid of sexual feelings is said to suffer from general sexual dysfunction. Typically she does not desire sex, and derives no sexual pleasure from erotic stimulation. In many instances she will exhibit little, if any, vaginal lubrication or swelling, but she may still engage in sexual activity due to concern for her sexual partner. On the other hand, she may actively avoid any type of sexual contact, even though she knows that the marital relationship will suffer as a result.

Primary general sexual dysfunction

A woman who has _never_ experienced sexual excitement, or erotic pleasure, with any partner, in any situation, displays the primary symptoms of this disorder. Psychological, organic, and/or situational factors may be involved.

Secondary general sexual dysfunction

A woman who presents the symptoms of general sexual dysfunction, having previously responded adequately to sexual stimulation, is said to have this secondary disorder. Sometimes these women responded well to premarital petting, but they became dysfunctional when the sexual stimulation escalated to coitus. Other women may be dysfunctional only in specific situations, or for isolated periods of time.

CHAPTER 5

Procedural Options for the Diagnosis and Treatment of Sexual Disorders

DIAGNOSIS

Differential Diagnosis

Diagnostic terminology

A sexual problem is clinically designated a sexual dysfunction when it disrupts, or evidences a disruption in, an individual's sexual response cycle. A sexual dysfunction can be either partial (an occasionally interrupted or a chronically weakened response) or complete (a total interruption). Those that have always existed are considered primary, while others that occur after a period of sexual adequacy, or situationally, are termed secondary. Dysfunctions are termed psychosexual or psychogenic when they are of emotional or social origin, while those that are organically precipitated are designated as secondary symptoms of the particular disease entity, for example, primary impotence, complete, secondary to chronic diabetes.

Diagnostic format

The differential diagnosis of a sexual complaint is established through the use of classical clinical procedures: the sexual history, physical examination, and mental status evaluation. When possible both partners should be included in this diagnostic format since sexual problems rarely arise apart from the sexual relationship.

Notes:

Diagnostic Procedures[1]

The sexual history

A thorough profile of each partner's sexual development, and a history of the sexual behavior within the relationship, is essential to the diagnosis and treatment of sexual disorders. Most clinicians (Hartman and Fithian, 1972; Kaplan, 1975; Masters and Johnson, 1970; and Shiller, 1973; etc.) agree that the therapist should combine a flexible, nonthreatening, indirect method of interviewing with a problem oriented approach. Wahl (1967), for example, recommends that the following general principles be kept in mind while taking a sex history:

1) Begin with those areas that are easily discussed before touching on the more difficult topics;

2) Identify how the patients initially obtained their sexual information before discussing their actual sexual experiences; and finally,

3) Whenever possible, "ubiquity statements" should be used to reassure patients as to the generality of either the experience or the information/misinformation. This latter technique is a good way to provide information while at the same time reducing shame, anxiety, and guilt.

Once the historical/developmental data has been obtained, the sexual complaint must be explored and delineated. Most sex therapists concur that the following information is an essential part of that clinical review:

1) How does the patient and his or her sexual partner perceive the problem? Who assigns blame? Who accepts blame? Are both partners willing to accept responsibility for their sexual relationship and enter therapy together? The possibility that the dysfunctional behavior may be offering some secondary gain must also be considered.

2) How long has the disorder been present? Is it a primary or

---

[1]Since most practicing clinicians are already familiar with these procedures, a detailed discussion has not been attempted here.

secondary dysfunction? Is it partial or complete, constant or intermittent?

3. <u>What were the emotional, social, and situational factors involved with the onset of the com-
plaint</u>? What else was going on when the first
symptoms occurred? Were there personal or em-
ployment problems?

4) <u>Does anything whatsoever diminish the sexual problem</u>? That is to say, has the patient found any way to bring about tempo-
rary or partial improvement in his or her
sexual functioning?

5) <u>Does the patient have an opinion as to the
etiology of the sexual disorder</u>?

6) <u>How serious does he or she think it is</u>?

7) <u>What are the patient's expectations regarding therapy</u>? Many seek treatment antici-
pating quick improvement through medication,
but are uncomfortable with psychotherapeutic
intervention.

Notes:

The medical evaluation

It is essential that sex therapists obtain
both a medical history and up-to-date medical information about those persons coming to them for
the treatment of sexual dysfunctions. This is
necessary so that a contributing organic disease,
physical problems, and/or pharmacologic factors
may be ruled out when they do not exist, or correctly identified and treated when they do.

The American Medical Association (1972, p.
17) has recommended that a complete physical examination "should precede treatment of every sexual complaint, regardless of the patient's sex."
Jon Meyer (1976) agrees with the A.M.A.'s position on this issue, and he emphasizes that a thorough examination of the genitals must be included in that procedure. Helen Kaplan, on the other hand, digresses from this traditional view
and recommends (1975) that a physical examination
(including medical laboratory tests[1]) be

---

[1]There is no standardized list of appropriate laboratory tests to be administered to sexually dysfunctional patients. One or more of the
following tests is often used, however, when the
examining physician suspects that he might indicate or rule out, organic involvement:

Notes:

conducted only when the sexual dysfunction, current physical symptoms, or the patient's medical
history indicates the necessity for it. This procedural flexibility is certainly commendable, but
it does not reduce the clinician's responsibility
to obtain comprehensive medical information about
the patient to aid in the establishment of an accurate diagnosis prior to embarking on any mode of
sex therapy.

The mental status evaluation

Because emotional factors can affect an individual's sexual functioning, it is important
that sex therapists have insight into the psychological make-up of both partners. Kaplan (1975)
notes that this is necessary so that they can:

(1) Determine the possible presence and
     nature of psychopathology in either
     sexual partner.

(2) Evaluate the quality of the couple's
     relationship, and

(3) Formulate an accurate impression
     of the role that the sexual symptom
     plays, intrapsychically, for each

Thyroxine studies (T_3T_4) for thyroid disease; a
Bromide Level to ascertain possible toxicity; a
three or five hour glucose tolerance test (GTT)
for blood sugar levels (this is essential with every impotent patient since diabetes is often the
cause of organic impotence); both the Veneral Disease Research Laboratory Test (VDRL) and a Gonorrhea Culture (GC) can be helpful in ruling out
possible neurological damage from veneral disease;
a Follicle Stimulating Hormone Analysis (FSH) and
an Estrogen Index Smear to determine hormone levels in women; and occasionally, a potassium hydro-
xide (KOH) preparation may be needed in diagnosing
fungal infections that could be involved in dyspareunia.

partner, and in their relationship.[1]

In some cases a brief psychiatric interview may be sufficient to disclose this type of
information; at other times, however, extensive
psychological testing could be indicated. When
the sex therapist is neither a psychiatrist nor
an extensively trained psychometrist it would be
appropriate to refer those patients who require
a more indepth approach.[2]

Diagnostic conclusions and implications for
treatment.

Once the sex history, medical and mental
status evaluations have been completed, a diagnosis should be evident and the implications for

---

[1]A 1959 study by Kleegman found that 85%
of the "frigid" women he treated were severely
neurotic, with only 15% manifesting "frigidity"
as a single symptom. Later, O'Connor and Stern
(1972) concluded that the psychiatric diagnosis
was a more important therapeutic/prognostic var-
iable than was sexual symptomatology itself.
Helen Kaplan (1974b) notes that the basic structure of the neurotic personality need not be
changed to correct sexual dysfunctions, but the
therapist must take these emotional conflicts
into account if the treatment is to be successful. Lobitz and LoPiccolo (1975), on the other
hand, imply that Kaplan does not go far enough,
and they recommend that the sex therapy modali-
ty be appropriately modified when patients evi-
dencing certain psychopathologies (depression,
obsessions, fear of loss of control, etc.) enter
treatment.

[2]In other cases, however, less sophisticated instruments can be used to obtain valuable
information important to sex therapy. For example, certain projective tests, such as the
graphic Draw-a-Person and the House-Tree-Person
test, etc., may conceivably be used even by the
not extensively psychometrically trained sex
therapist, just as other nonpsychometrists regularly use self-rating devices such as Zung's
Depression Scale (Zung, 1965, 1967a, 1967b, 1967c,
1973; Zung, Richards & Short, 1965), Popoff's
Index of Depression (Popoff, 1969a, 1969b), the
Cornell Medical Index (1949), the ROCOM Health
History (1971), and various personality question
naires (e.g., Annon's Sexual Fear Inventory, 1975b,
1975c; Pion's Sexual Response Profile, 1975; and
Robinson and Annon's Heterosexual Behavior Inventory, 1975a. 1975b). Any of these instruments,
and others similar to them, can be used in or
easily adapted to the sex therapy setting.

Notes:

treatment should be clear. If the sexual disorder is medically based, then it must be treated as a medical problem -- rather than a sexual dysfunction -- even though there may be sexual symptoms. This is also true for sexual problems that are secondary to psychiatric disorders; in these cases psychotherapy, or other types of psychiatric care, may be indicated. If, on the other hand, the dysfunctional behavior is an emotionally based learned disorder, arising out of ignorance, or from a troubled relationship, it is termed psychogenic, and frequently the dysfunctional symptoms can be relieved by the short-term psychotherapeutic/educational techniques that have been developed to treat psychosexual dysfunctions.

TREATMENT

Once the etiology of the sexual disorder has been established, treatment can begin. Often psychogenic sexual problems can be successfully treated by simple sex education; not infrequently, however, relationship counseling and psychotherapy are also required. On those occasions when educational and/or counseling procedures prove insufficient to remove or satisfactorily diminish the sexual symptom it may be necessary to shift one's clinical approach to include certain experiential, behaviorially desensitizing procedures (termed sexual "tasks," "exercises," or "homework assignments") that can help reduce the disruptive sexual anxiety to a level where it is possible for the dysfunctional partner to relearn adequate sexual responses.

Sex Education and Counseling[1]

Sex Education

Many sexual problems are the result of ignorance. Sex education is, therefore, one of the treatment techniques most widely used by sex therapists. Often, simple straightforward infor-

_____

[1]Practicing clinicians should be familiar with most of these techniques; therefore, their application has not been discussed here at great length. As will be shown in the next chapter, however, all of these procedures are important to the psychotherapeutic treatment of psychosexual dysfunction, so they have been included here along with a more thorough discussion of those other techniques and procedures (e.g., sensate focus exercises) that are virtually unique to sex therapy, and which may be unfamiliar to many clinical professionals.

mation about human sexual behavior can correct inappropriate expectations and/or wrong assumptions, while providing a foundation for improved, more adequate sexual functioning (Jankovich and Miller, 1978).

Sometimes, however, sexual ignorance may be only part of the problem. In these cases educational techniques (films, books, etc.) must be combined with other clinical procedures (counseling, behavioral training, etc.) so as to create a comprehensive treatment approach to the sexual disorder.

The sexual information examination

When the sex history reveals, or the therapist suspects, that the sexual disorder is a result of the couple's ignorance of sexual anatomy, or to profound sexual anxiety associated with personal nudity, it may prove helpful to order a "sexological" or sexual information examination.[1] This educational procedure, which consists of an examination of the genitalia, and other erotically sensitive areas, is performed by a medical clinician on each partner, both individually and in the presence of the other. The following description by Kirker and Kirker (1980)[2] is illustrative of the procedure:

> We employ the following procedure on all couples being treated for sexual dysfunction. The aim of this examination is twofold: to provide sexual information and to evaluate the couple's response during an anxiety-provoking situation.

> At the start of counseling, the co-therapists explain to the couple

---

[1]The sexual information examination should not be confused with the diagnostic medical evaluation which also requires a physical examination. They are distinctly separate procedures that are undertaken for different clinical reasons.

[2]In their description of this clinical procedure, Kirker and Kirker utilize the male-female co-therapist approach pioneered by Masters and Johnson. Such a format is not essential to the success of the procedure, however, and it is regularly employed by medically trained sex therapists practicing alone (Croft, 1975).

Notes:

that the first part of the treatment
will be a physical examination conducted jointly by the co-therapists
and the couple in therapy.

On the day of the examination, the
couple is ushered into the consultation room. The co-therapists and the
couple discuss various sexual attitudes
such as body image, nudity, and
myths surrounding sexual activity.
After ten or fifteen minutes of discussion, one member of the couple is
escorted to an examination room and
is instructed to undress completely,
put on a gown, and sit on the examination table. The other partner and
the co-therapists enter the room for
the physical examination.

Examination of the female partner is
carried out in the following manner.
The female co-therapist (a certified
nurse practitioner) proceeds with a
general, non-threatening examination
of the eyes, ears, mouth, and listen-
ing to the heart and lungs. The patient is then asked to lie down. The
female co-therapist examines the
breasts and discusses the breast
engorgement and nipple changes that
occur during sexual excitement, and
the sexual blush. The therapist
points out other erotic areas of
the body, such as the neck, ears,
and thighs. An abdominal examination follows, with discussion of
female and male body hair distribution.

In preparation for a pelvic examination, the head of the table is raised,
and the woman positions her feet in
the stirrups. A hand mirror is given
to the patient, in order that she may
view her own genitalia. The male partner is instructed to sit beside the female therapist for close observation
and participation during the examination.

The female therapist conducts the
pelvic examination. She examines and
describes the anatomical features of
the vulva, including the inner thighs,
labia minora and majora, and clitoris.
She discusses completely the changes
that occur in the external genitalia

during sex. Special emphasis is
given to the clitoris and its
role in female orgasmic response.
The male partner is asked to ex-
amine the clitoris.

A Graves bi-valve vaginal speculum is inserted into the vagina. A
fibro-optic light is attached to
the speculum for better viewing.
Both partners observe the vagina,
cervix and cervical os while the
therapist gives an anatomical description. After receiving instructions from the female therapist, the male partner takes a Pap smear.

Slowly and gently, the female
therapist removes the speculum from
the vagina. As the speculum is
being removed, the adaptability
of the vagina to containment is
verified. The examination is over,
and the woman is asked to dress.
This examination usually takes
about thirty minutes.

The role of the male therapist,
during the examination of the female patient, is one of observer.
He closely follows the behavior
of the couple during the examination, making mental notes of such
reactions as embarrassment, anxiety, or disinterest, for discussion at a later time.

Examination of the male partner is carried out in the following manner. The man is instructed to undress, put on a gown, and
sit upon the examination table.
The female partner and the co-
therapists enter the room. The
male therapist begins with the
desensitizing physical examination of the head, neck, throat,
heart, lungs and blood pressure.
The female partner is encouraged
to participate throughout the
examination. The female
therapist acts as an observer,
making mental notes of the couple's reactions, for future discussion.

While the male partner is lying down, the male therapist

Notes:

Notes:

describes again and re-emphasizes the
sexual aspects of the breasts, nipples
and other erogenous zones. The genitalia are then exposed, with an anatomical
discussion of male sexual response.
The female partner is then encouraged to palpate the testicles, vas de-
ferens and inguinal canal. The therapist describes and demonstrates the
"squeeze technique" and then the female partner practices the technique.

To complete the physical, the male
therapist performs a rectal examination, to check the prostate gland.

This examination takes approximately twenty to twenty-five minutes.

After the completion of both examinations, the couple and the co-therapists return to the conference room,
where the four discuss openly their
thoughts and feelings about the exam-
ations.

This educational procedure, which was intro-
duced to sex therapists by Hartman and Fithian (1972,
pp. 77-98), is now widely used in the treatment of
psychogenic sexual dysfunction. Croft (1975), therefore, seemingly speaks for many sex therapists when
he notes that the sexual information examination is
an excellent clinical tool because it is helpful in:

1) Exposing sexual myths and misconceptions,

2) Giving permission,

3) Desensitizing (or increasing comfort),

4) Building rapport, and in some cases,

5) shortening the duration of therapy.

Psychotherapy

The resolution of conflicts is often essential to the successful treatment of psychosexual dysfunctions. Realizing this, sex therapists have
included psychotherapeutic procedures into their
treatment formats. The distinguishing characteristic of these psychotherapeutic approaches, however,
is that they limit their scope to the conflicts associated with the particular sexual disorder, and
they intervene only to the point necessary for the
individual's sexual responses to function adequately.

Relationship counseling

Marriage counseling, or couples therapy, is
often indicated when sexual problems develop.
This is so because sexual disorders can be sympto-
matic of conflicts present within the relationship
(Racy, 1977). When this is the case, and the relationship goes untreated, not only can the sexual dysfunction become chronic, but it also becomes another point of conflict, thus compounding
the already troubled situation (Mann and Katsuranis,
1975).

At other times, when the dysfunction occurs
as a symptom of other factors (pressures at work,
financial problems, etc.), various negative pressures may still be exerted on the relationship.
If this stress is sufficient to damage communication within the relationship, it is likely that
additional conflicts will result, and the previously healthy relationship may be even more
threatened (Fay, 1977).

Sex therapists must always remember that
psychosexual dysfunctions do not exist in isolation from a sexual relationship, and they must
take great care to understand how certain relational factors may be causing, compounding, or aggra-
vating the sexual symptom. These factors must
then be taken into account and dealt with directly. To do otherwise would be to ignore clinical
data that are often vital to the successful treatment of dysfunctional sexual behavior.

Sex Therapy

The psychotherapeutic/experiential approach

Sexual dysfunctions are often a part of, or
the result of very complex intrapsychic and social
mechanisms. When, after a suitable trial period,
the more elementary approaches of sex education
and counseling are not able to bring about or restore adequate sexual functioning when employed a-
lone, it may become necessary to incorporate into
the treatment program the experiential (or behav-
iorial) technique of in vivo desensitization. Naturally each sexual dysfunction may require its
own distinct desensitizing procedure or variation,
and each sex therapist will probably contribute
certain clinical approaches or treatment techniques
that are unique. Regardless of these idiosyncra-
sies, however, one particular procedure (the "sensate focus" or "sexual pleasuring exercise") has
been shown to have such universal clinical applica-
bility that it is widely used in the treatment of a
variety of psychogenic sexual dysfunctions.

Notes:

The sensate focus, "pleasuring" exercise

Helen Kaplan (1975) attributes Masters and Johnson with "inventing" the term sensate focus for the pleasuring exercise they pioneered at the Reproductive Biology Research Foundation in St. Louis. Basically, when a couple is assigned this pleasuring task, they are asked to refrain from coitus and orgasm for a period that might last from several days to several weeks. During this time they are asked to set aside moments when they can gently massage or caress each other in a nondemanding, accepting way.

Non-Genital Pleasuring

In the very beginning of this part of the therapy non-genital pleasuring may be prescribed. Sometimes, when sexual anxiety is very high, or when the couple's relationship has significantly deteriorated, the sex therapist may even order that the sensate focus exercise begin with one partner caressing only the hand of the other. This allows for physical contact to begin with the least possible sexual threat. Later, as the couple becomes more comfortable with this type of contact, the therapist will ask that they become increasingly more intimate, eventually requiring that their pleasuring exercise include other parts of their bodies -- the face, feet, and shoulders. Ideally, the patients will become so comfortable with the sensate focus massage that they will at some point be able to tolerate, and even enjoy, a fully nude, total body caress.

Genital Pleasuring

With genital pleasuring the goal is that the patients should learn to produce and respond to sexual arousal.[1] (Arousal to the point of orgasm, however, remains forbidden.) For some, this will be an opportunity to have their initial experience with comfortable genital intimacy and sexual arousal, while for others, genital pleasuring will simply be the vehicle by which this lost comfort is restored.

As the couple experiences sexual arousal

---

[1]Variations on genital pleasuring, such as the squeeze technique, dilatation, and self-stimulation, will be described and discussed later when their appropriate clinical application can be thoroughly explained.

through genital intimacy they are encouraged to focus on their reactions -- that is, on those feelings which this behavior engenders: anxiety, guilt, boredom, pleasure, etc. These feelings then become the central focus of the sex therapy experience, and their effective clarification/resolution is the clinical task for both the therapist and the patients.

Reactions

Most couples have positive responses to the non-genital pleasuring: "It was nice, I really enjoyed it"; "I love a deep massage but [the sexual partner] would never do it before," or simply, "It was very relaxing." Sometimes, however, even these very elementary attempts at physical intimacy are so threatening that they may provoke negative responses; when this happens the defense mechanisms of avoidance ("We just didn't have time to do it") or sabotage ("It was so boring that I just couldn't do it -- besides, it's such a silly exercise") are often employed to maintain the status quo.

Similar responses occur as a result of genital pleasuring, but as Kaplan (1975) points out, a specific type of emotional reaction evidences itself here: sexual anxiety. Naturally, this affective response can be to any degree, from very mild ("It didn't do much for me") to severe ("I can't stand him doing that; why the hell do people have to have sex, anyway!"), but its presence indicates the existence of conflict (intrapsychic, marital, social, or religious, etc.) which must be dealt with before therapy can continue.

Rationale

The reason this sexual pleasuring exercise works so well is not clearly understood. Most probably it is due to a combination of many factors that can be described in various ways and understood differently, depending on one's theoretical/clinical perspective.

Obviously, the behavioral learning components of the sensate focus exercise are important to its clinical success. That is to say, the mandatory prohibition against both coitus and orgasm interrupts the sequence of habitually inadequate sexual responses; the non-genital pleasuring then lowers the anxiety that had been previously associated with intimate physical contact. The genital caresses subsequently teach both partners that sexual arousal can be

Notes:

pleasurable and rewarding, and the dysfunctional patients are then able to learn sexually adequate responses and give up their previously inadequate behaviors.

During this same period, of course, the therapist works to clarify other factors (intrapsychic conflict, relational problems and social/professional/religious issues, etc.) that could also be involved in producing the dysfunctional symptom. This means, then, that in addition to the behavioral rationale, psychoanalytic theory and marital dynamics are also structured into the therapy setting. Therefore, no one system, theory, or clinical approach, can be singularly credited with success.

Variations in the clinical application of therapeutic options.

Naturally, there are a variety of approaches to the clinical treatment of psychosexual **dysfunctions, and all sex therapists are encouraged to** be both flexible and creative when they translate therapeutic technique from theory into practice. For example, a classical treatment procedure recommended by such experts as Masters and Johnson, Kaplan, Meyer, and/or others, may not be suitable, or its effects may not be sufficiently long-lasting in particular situations, or with a certain couple. This should not suggest, however, that the sexual dysfunction presented under these circumstances is untreatable; it simply means that the sex therapist will have to develop new procedures, or redesign old ones, so that they can be usefully applied in the particular situation. This type of creativity is illustrated in the following case report:

A thirty-three-year-old white female informed her physician that she was pre-orgasmic (i.e. primary nonorgasmia). She also complained of depressive feelings and almost a complete lack of sexual desire. Unfortunately, the patient absolutely refused referral to a sex therapist because her husband (also a physician) had told her "they are all quacks."
Since she refused referral, her doctor decided to treat her himself, with the combination of a tricyclic antidepressant and masturbation training. (This approach, while certainly not widely employed, has been established as a viable clinical option through the research and reporting

of D.C. Renshaw, 1974 and 1975.)

The patient was placed on Doxepin HCL, 100 mg. h.s. for two weeks; at that point her dosage was increased to 150 mg. h.s. During this time she was also instructed to masturbate, by herself, daily -- during or after her bath, when she would be most relaxed. (Coitus was also proscribed, but she doubted that her husband would notice because he had stopped approaching her for sex play since she had refused almost all of his advances during the previous six months.)

After three weeks on this combination of treatments the patient noted a "lift" in her mood and a "mild" increase in her sexual desire. During the fourth week, on her own initiative, she began masturbating twice daily -- once after her husband left for work in the morning, and again during her bath at mid-afternoon.

By the end of the fifth week she reported that she and her husband were getting along better (this was seen as resulting from her improved affect), and her sexual desire was much stronger (also probably due to the antidepressant effects of the Doxepin HCL). Orgasm still eluded her, however, but she was now "even more determined" to experience that sensation.

This reward was not long in coming. On her next visit to her physician, the following week, she glowingly acknowledged that she had been twice orgasmic, due to masturbation, while bathing. She was then asked to continue her masturbation, but she was now encouraged to also share these experiences with her husband. Later, that same week, she called her doctor and reported that she had finally been orgasmic with cunnilingus. [Crist, 1980].

Clearly, then, both creativity and flexibility are valuable assets to those clinicians undertaking treatment of sexual disorders. For when neither tradition nor established clinical theory are sufficient, the clinician's only other resources are his or her own professional expertise and informed ingenuity.

CHAPTER 6

The Application of Procedural Options for the Diagnosis and Treatment of Sexual Disorders

Sexual inadequacies can occur for many reasons. This means that no single diagnostic perspective or treatment approach can be expected to fit every need. Nevertheless, certain perspectives and approaches have met with repeated clinical success, and they are outlined in this chapter.

MALE SEXUAL DYSFUNCTIONS

Impotence

A male who is unable to obtain or maintain an erection, sufficient to satisfactorily complete sexual intercourse, is impotent (Levine, 1976b). Primary impotence[1] is indicated when such erection has never occurred; secondary impotence is the term which characterizes an erectile dysfunction that has occurred after a period of adequate sexual functioning.

Diagnosis

Sexual history

Once the primary or secondary nature of the erectile failure has been established, the therapist must determine the degree of residual erective capacity. For example, is the dysfunctional response partial (either unfirm or not

---

[1] Primary impotence is rare, but Taylor (1975) notes that there have been occasional reports of its occurring due to "congenital testicular dysfunction, such as Klinefelter's syndrome, in which the hormonal balance is clearly at fault" (p. 740).

Notes:

sufficiently long-lasting) or _complete_? Is it _con_-stant or _episodic_? Does it occur _situationally_ (only at home, or just when he is very tired, etc.), _selectively_ (with his wife, but not with prostitutes, or during masturbation), or _generally_?

After these characteristics have been noted, a clear profile of each partner, and the relationship, should be created. For example, were their earliest experiences with sexual activity positive, or did they learn that sex was dirty? Under what circumstances did they first experience genital contact? Was it a good experience, or did it produce fear, guilt, etc.? What is the condition of their relationship? How sensitive are they to each other? Do they understand and accept their own, and each other's sexual needs and limitations.

Next, the therapist should explore each partner's reaction to the erectile disorder, and the role that it has played in, or the effect it has had on, the relationship. For instance, under what circumstances did impotence first occur? How did he respond to it? What was her reaction? Has their relationship been seriously affected because of it? If so, how?

This information can then be drawn together into an interpretive statement that should shed some light on the etiology and perpetuation of the erectile dysfunction. For example, the man may have been under great stress, or very fatigued, during the period when it initially occurred. His wife, having felt neglected because of his lack of attention during that same period, resented this additional -- failure which she perceived as further neglect -- and reacted negatively. Her husband then panicked, fearing that she may begin to have doubts about his masculinity, but this additional stress created such anxiety that his subsequent attempts were also without success. His wife then became even more frustrated ("What's the matter with you?"); he interpreted those feelings as rejection, and they became even more estranged -- making successful coitus virtually impossible.

Sometimes, of course, the sex history will indicate that neither developmental nor relational factors were directly involved in the erectile dysfunction. This may be the case when both partners are emotionally mature and secure in themselves and in their relationship, and when outside factors (debts, problems at work, etc.) can be seen to create _feelings of failure_ in the male -- feelings which he then acts out in his sex life.

Essentially, his inadequate sexual response may be
expressing a more generalized feeling of inadequacy that he has developed because of repeated professional or financial failures; but
even in these cases, the **developmental/relational**
material must be covered because nothing can be
ruled out unless information about it is first
obtained, and then evaluated. Likewise, to determine the extent of organic and/or psychiatric
involvement, if any, a thorough physical examination is required, and a mental status evaluation may be necessary -- if so indicated by
the sex history or other material.

Notes:

Medical evaluation

Impotence is a symptom indicating an interruption in the excitement phase of the male's
sexual response cycle; usually ejaculation is not
affected if the flaccid penis can be sufficiently
stimulated. In 85 - 90% of these cases the interruption is of a psychogenic nature; but the
fact that 10 - 15% of all impotent patients have
some organic or pharmacologic involvement suggests
that a thorough medical history, physical examination, and some laboratory tests should be undertaken with each patient complaining of erectile
failure (Renshaw, 1978).

Psychiatric/psychological evaluation

Various psycho-sexual factors can bring on
psychogenic impotence. Masters and Johnson
(1970) note that the seven most common causes
are: religious orthodoxy, efforts to control a
prior state of premature ejaculation, alcoholic
intake, depreciation of the male role and status,
homosexual orientation, marital disharmony, and
cultural pressure to perform sexually. Domeena
Renshaw (1978) expands this list to include anxiety, anger, depression, the "madonna complex",[1]
and the absence of sexually arousing materials
or actions (e.g., fetish objects, spanking,
binding, etc.). Boyarsky and Boyarsky (1978), on
the other hand, narrow the clinical focus and
identify only one major psychological cause of
impotence: fear.

Whenever the sex therapist believes -- or

---

[1]The "madonna complex" is described by
Renshaw (1978) as "a cultural attitude held by
some men that sex is 'dirty' and to be done only
with 'loose women' not with wives who are also
mothers...these men fear that lust may contamin-

Notes:

even suspects -- that these or other psycho-social factors are playing an important part in the etiology of the erectile dysfunction, a mental status evaluation is recommended. In some cases this may require only a limited psychiatric interview, while at other times formal psychological testing may be necessary.

Diagnostic conclusions

If the medical evaluation uncovers organic or pharmacologic involvement, the precipitating condition will require medical attention. Sometimes this will necessitate only a minor adjustment in the patient's prescribed medication (Serafetinides, 1972), or a recommendation that he limit his alcohol consumption (Farkas and Rosen, 1976), and adequate sexual functioning may rapidly return; at other times, however, more dramatic steps might be needed. For example, when the erectile disorder has been brought on by advanced diabetes, the neurologic damage may be so severe that normal erection will never again be possible even after the disease has been medically controlled. In some of these cases the surgical implantation of a penile prosthesis may be the treatment of choice (Furlow, 1976; Kent, 1975; Osborne, 1976; Sethnoy and Roy, 1976). In other instances, however, the couple may only require sex education to broaden their sexual horizons so that other types of erotic intimacy will be available to them since penile/vaginal intercourse is no longer a viable option (Kales, et al., 1977).

When the medical evaluation rules out both organic and pharmacological factors, as it most often will, sex education and counseling may be helpful in reducing or reversing the dysfunctional behavior. Sometimes, for example, sex education can erase unrealistic performance expectations, and restore adequate sexual functioning in just a short time. In other cases individual psychotherapy or relationship counseling may be necessary to help reduce stress and resolve conflicts that have prevented adequate sexual responses in the past. When these options, employed either individually or in various combinations, are not successful, however, it may be advantageous to introduce certain behavioral sex therapy techniques that can facilitate treatment.

Treatment: Sex Education and Counseling

Sex education

Both partners should be given accurate information pertaining to the anatomy, physiology, and psychology of sexual functioning, especially erectile response. This will not only help to reduce the flood of anxiety produced by sexual ignorance which is often the cause of psychogenic impotence, but it can also provide them with a framework that will allow them to more reasonably appraise their own sexual expectations and performances.

The couple should be told, for instance, that approximately half the male population has at one time or another experienced transient episodes of impotence, and they should understand that such occasional failures fall within the limits of normal sexual behavior. They should also learn that when a man is tired or worried or depressed, it may take much more sexual stimulation to arouse him, and sometimes -- if his preoccupation is complete -- arousal to erection is for the moment impossible. Furthermore, they should be informed about the effects of alcohol on penile response,[1] and how marital disharmony can upset just about any type of sexual functioning.

Information of this nature is often helpful to the treatment of psychogenic impotence because it provides the couple with a foundation from which they can more realistically appraise their own sexual expectations and functioning. This not only reduces anxiety, but in many cases it tends to improve sexual performance. Moreover, because each partner is then more knowledgeable about sexual functioning, they are better prepared to modify their own behaviors (e.g., a decision to reduce alcohol consumption prior to coitus) so that they can avoid similar episodes in the future.

Sexual information examination

Anxiety about sexual activity, reproduction, and/or the genitalia may have a significant effect on the male's ability to function adequately as a coital partner. For example, if he has been taught that sex is dirty and that the genitals are unclean, or if he does not feel secure with the contraception he and his partner are practicing, he may unconsciously protect himself

Notes:

---

[1]In their 1976 study, Farkas and Rosen found that large doses of alcohol depressed both penile diameter increase and tumescence rate. From this data they concluded that erectile depression, such as that produced by alcohol, can prevent the formation or maintenance of an erection suitable for vaginal penetration. Moreover, "excessive drinking may be an important etiological factor in certain cases of male impotence" (p. 271).

Notes:

from future sexual contact through impotence.
In cases such as these a sexological examination
can be helpful -- when used as part of a comprehensive educational/counseling approach to
treatment -- because it can initiate a basic
level of sexual/genital desensitization, and it
can serve as the beginning point from which the
therapeutic process can branch out to include all
areas of human sexual intimacy.

Psychotherapy

In cases where the erectile inhibition has
been precipated (primarily) by severe intrapsychic
conflicts, brief directive psychotherapy may be
called for. In fact, Kent (1975) implies that
psychogenic impotence can be successfully managed
using only psychotherapy and instruction in sexual technique. Lording (1978) also values the psychotherapeutic approach, noting that in males who
present with their first episode of impotence,
which is of short duration, and with an identifi-
able precipitating factor, the prognosis -- using
simple psychotherapy -- is really quite good (i.e.,
the resolution of impotence in over two thirds of
the patients treated): "The principles involved
include an attempt to reduce performance pressure
by de-emphasizing sexual intercourse as the goal of
all sexual activities, and to provide information
and counseling about sexual function and behavior.
The therapist need not be a psychiatrist" (p. 149).
Most often, however, psychotherapeutic intervention serves as only a part of a total treatment
approach which may also include basic sex education,
relationship counseling, and even behavioral desensitization.

Relationship counseling

When psychological impotence is not the result
of intrapsychic conflict, it is due to problems within the relationship (Goldberg, 1972). This point is
highlighted by Levine (1976b) who states that impotence due to interpersonal factors usually sig-
nals profound partner alienation and a severely deteriorated relationship.

The patient may recount his wife's de-
ficies; their fights; the cold,
silent interactions; the infidelity,
and thoughts of divoce. Even without such obvious evidence, his sarcas-
tic, bitter, accusatory, or coldly in-
different tone conveys the lack of affection. His undistrubed potency before the relationship deterioration

completes the pattern of erectile
dysfunction due to interpersonal
causes [p. 345].

In cases where psychogenic impotence has been
precipitated by partner alienation or because of
a severe deterioration of the relationship, conjoint relationship counseling will be an essential part of any treatment program (Graber and Kline-
Graber, 1977), even if sex education, individual
psychotherapy, and/or behavioral sex therapy approaches are also utilized. Indeed, it is very
unlikely that adequate sexual functioning could
reoccur -- on a lasting basis -- in a relationship that is characterized by anger and mistrust
(Fogarty, 1977).

Treatment: Sex Therapy

Both sex education and counseling can be
very helpful in the treatment of psychogenic impotence, but frequently they must be supplemented
by certain behavioral treatment techniques that
focus directly on the erectile inadequacy.

Prohibitions and prescriptions

Before sex therapy actually begins, the
clinician must establish that both partners are
committed to the therapeutic goal (potency);
otherwise, it is unlikely that genuine progress
will be made.[1] Next, the couple must agree to
postpone indefinitely all recreational coital interaction so that further reinforcement of the
dysfunctional behavior does not occur. Finally,
each must be willing and able to regularly practice the sexual tasks that have been designed to
shape a more adequate erectile response: often
this will require some modifications in their
work or social schedules during the entire period of therapy.

Sensate focus

Typically, the sensate focus sexual pleasuring exercise is initiated at the start of therapy. The couple begins by doing daily non-genital pleasuring and continues with this type of
light, nondemanding massage until they feel

Notes:

---

[1]Sometimes the secondary gain from the dysfunctional behavior will be so important (for
one or both of the partners) that treatment will
be repeatedly sabotaged. When this occurs both
relationship counseling and/or individual psychotherapy may be necessary prerequisites to sex
the-

Notes:

comfortable with such physical intimacy, and are
prepared to move on to sexually arousing genital
contact. Nondemand genital pleasuring is then practiced on a daily basis until the male naturally
responds with erection. (It is recommended that
orgasm be postponed so that he can be restimulated
to erection several times during a short period;
his repeated success at achieving erection is
very therapeutic.)

Extravaginal ejaculation

Once the male has gained confidence in his
own potency, the genital pleasuring progresses
to extravaginal orgasm. This may occur by either
manual or oral stimulation.

Vaginal containment

By this time the male should feel quite
comfortable with his ability to achieve and maintain erection, and to ejaculate extravaginally
due to erotic stimulation. He is then ready to
experience vaginal containment. This is simply a
continuation of the same arousing exercises practiced before, with the exception that the erect
penis is finally inserted into the vagina. Pelvic
thrusting may then occur, but only extravaginal
ejaculation should be permitted. (This restric-
tion will be modified in the next phase of therapy, but at this point it serves to protect the
male from undue anxiety brought on by premature
performance expectations.)

Intravaginal ejaculation

In this last stage of therapy the final prohibition is removed. He is told that he may now
ejaculate intravaginally, if he chooses, but it
is also made clear that this is not a requirement.
He is thus set free to experience coitus as he
wishes -- without any limitations or expectations.

Results of Treatment

Masters and Johnson (1970) report dramatically fewer failures when treating secondary erectile dysfunction (26.3%) than with primary impotence (40.6%). They offer no concrete reasons
for this, but one might infer that primary sexual
dysfunctions are almost always more difficult to
"cure."

Helen Kaplan (1974b) notes similar experiences in her work with erectile dysfunction.

Preliminary evidence...suggests that

> when secondary impotence occurs in a
> man who is reasonably healthy other-
> wise, it has an excellent prognosis...
>
> Primary impotence has a less favorable
> prognosis...Yet it is also frequently
> response to the brief treatment pro-
> cedure [p. 287].

Despite the variety of successes that these
and other sex therapists have reported, it must
be pointed out that the "cure" is not always long-
lasting. Masters and Johnson (1970, p. 367) report
a 5% relapse rate among those patients treated
for impotence, at the time of their five-year
follow-up. Kaplan (1974b) also reports a "modest"
amount of relapse among her patients, but she
quotes no specific figures. Very striking data
are offered by Levine and Agle (1978), however,
who report that, in one controlled study, "during
the follow-up year...only 1 out of 16 chronically
impotent men maintained the high level of success
achieved by the end of therapy" (p. 245).

In commenting on the possible reasons for
the frequency of relapse back into impotence,
Kaplan (1974b) alludes to various interpersonal
factors, and notes that the return of the erectile
disorder may be due to a dramatic deterioration
in the patient's relationship with his partner.
Levine and Agle (1978) evaluate the situation differently, however. They focus their attention on
the treatment procedures themselves and suggest
that brief sex therapy -- as it is now understood
and practiced -- is only effective in improving
erectile functioning (p. 249), and that is inappropriate to expect it to "restore complete sexual
health to couples with this complicated disorder"
(p. 235).

This high level of relapse among patients
treated for impotence is certainly disturbing.
Nevertheless, it must be kept in mind that the re-
lapsed patient should be again amenable to sex
therapy, and it may be that these subsequent treatments will proceed more quickly and produce somewhat longer lasting results than did the initial
experience.

Premature Ejaculation

It is not at all uncommon for couples to
complain that their ejaculation is "too fast," but
sometimes it is difficult to determine whether this
lack of ejaculatory control is of dysfunctional

Notes: proportions.[1] Perhaps the best guideline for establishing this is offered by the therapists at
the Cornell Medical Center (Kaplan et al., 1974)
who define premature ejaculation as "the inability of a man to tolerate high (plateau) levels of
sexual excitement without ejaculating reflexly"
(p. 444).

Diagnosis

Sexual history

Initially, the sex therapist must establish
a clear description of the sexual disorder. For
example, how long have the dysfunctional symptoms
existed? Are they primary (very rare) or secondary?
Partial or complete? Constant or episodic? Situational, selective, or general?

Then, because a variety of social/sexual
learning situations can set the stage for premature
ejaculation, it is necessary to obtain a thorough
sexual history of both individuals and the sexual
relationship. For example, it could be that his
masturbation was always under hurried circumstances
("Why are you taking so long in the bathroom?"),
or that his early sexual experiences required
great speed (which is often the case when these occasions were "rushed" -- on dates, or with prostitutes, etc.), with the result that he has never
learned that it is permissable for him to "take
his time." On the other hand, if -- during coitus
-- his present sexual partner frequently complains
that "it hurts" (dyspareunia), it might be that he
is unconsciously (but intentionally) terminating
the sex act so that he will no longer be responsible for causing her pain.

Nonsexual factors must also be taken into account during the sex history. For instance,

---

[1]Wabrek and Wabrek (1977) state that premature ejaculation is the most common male sexual dysfunction found in our society. Interestingly, this
"common" male sexual dysfunction has not yet been
precisely defined, nor is there wide agreement a-
mong sex therapists as to its specific symptoms
(cf. Kaplan, 1974b; Kaplan et al., 1974; Levine,
1975, 1976a; LoPiccolo and Lobitz, 1972; Masters
and Johnson, 1970; Meyer, 1976; O'Connor and Stern,
1972; and O'Connor, 1976). This means that there
are no universally accepted clinical criteria for
distinguishing between fast, very fast, and dysfunc-
tionally premature ejaculatory responses.

persons who work under the stress of "get it done
on time" (sales, reports, production quotas, etc.)
may also carry this expectation/response into
their bedrooms. Indeed, if they have been trained
to "work quickly" on the job, it is not unlikely
that they will respond similarly elsewhere.

Therefore, to obtain an accurate profile of
the psychological/social factors that may be involved in the etiology of premature ejaculation,
sex therapists must not only obtain a detailed description of the dysfunctional symptoms as they
appear in the sexual relationship, and a thorough
developmental sexual history of each sexual partner, but they must also attempt to piece together
an accurate behavioral/social profile of the dysfunctional partner. This information can then be
used to clarify the specifics of the sexual complaint, and to suggest further diagnostic approaches -- medical, psychological, etc.

Medical evaluation

Cases of organically based premature ejaculation are extremely rare. This notwithstanding,
a thorough medical examination (possibly including a
urological and a neurological evaluation) may be indicated when the prematurity is of sudden onset. In
such cases, the symptom of quick ejaculation may be
indicative of serious illness. Helen Kaplan notes
that, although such cases are very infrequent, premature ejaculation may be caused by "local disease
of the posterior urethra, e.g., prostatitis. Or,
...secondary ejaculatory incontinence may be symptom-
atic of pathology along the nerve pathways subserv-
ing the reflex mechanisms which control orgasm --
in the spinal cord, peripheral nerves, or higher
nervous centers" (1974b, p. 293).

Naturally, when the sexual history reveals
that the female partner is experiencing physical
pain during coitus (dyspareunia), she must also
receive a thorough physical examination. It could
be that she is suffering from sexual/medical problems that are precipitating or compounding her
partner's dysfunctional behavior.

Psychiatric/psychological evaluation

If the sexual, social, or medical histories
suggest that emotional problems (acute anxiety,
phobias, obsessive-compulsive disorders, etc.)
may be evident, a thorough psychiatric evaluation
is required. In some cases a routine M.M.P.I.
can be helpful in either diagnosing or ruling out
psychiatric problems.

Notes:

Notes:

Diagnostic conclusions

If organic factors are involved, they must be treated medically. Usually, however, anxiety, unrealistic performance expectations, problems of intimacy, and/or a history of "quickness" bring on premature ejaculation. In these cases -- when the cause is psychogenic -- sex education, counseling/psychotherapy, and sex therapy are the treatments of choice.

Treatment: Sex Education and Counseling

Sex education

Treatment begins with a discussion of sexual behavior which focuses on the ejaculatory response. For some couples this will be the only treatment they require. Indeed, insightful persons who are able to exert a reasonable amount of control over their own lives and behavior may be able to "slow down" once they understand the dynamics of their dysfunction. For others, however, sex education (discussion, books, movies, etc.) will only be the beginning of treatment.

Sexual information examination

In some males, premature ejaculation may not only indicate an ignorance of sexual behavior and response, but it may also suggest some discomfort with -- and/or ignorance of -- sexual anatomy. This is often the case with young males who may ejaculate immediately upon vaginal penetration or soon thereafter. For these persons, and their sexual partners, the sexological examination can be a very helpful educational/desensitizing technique.

Psychotherapy

When the sexual history or the psychiatric evaluation suggests that the prematurity is the result of unresolved conflicts, psychotherapy may be necessary. Most often, however, psychotherapeutic treatment will not be, in and of itself, sufficient to completely reverse the dysfunctional ejaculatory response and certain sex therapy procedures will still be required.

Relationship counseling

Often a sexual inadequacy is indicative of a deteriorating relationship and the sexual dysfunction is itself the characteristic symptom, or sign, of those missing feelings of warmth and

trust. Sometimes, for example, an alienated wife's
hostile, demanding attitude may precipitate anxious and insecure feelings within her spouse. He
reacts to this stress by ejaculating too quickly
which alienates her even more, and their problems
are perpetuated. At other times, however, premature ejaculation may directly point to an angry male's need "to misuse his wife, to disdain-
fully disregard her wishes, and to frustrate her
sexual aspirations" (Levine, 1976a, p. 576). In
either case, relationship counseling will be an essential part of treatment since it is unlikely
that any significant delay in such ejaculatory
responses can be achieved without first removing
the major obstacles of conflict, and then restoring a reasonable level of trust conducive to intimacy.

Treatment: Sex Therapy

When ejaculation cannot be satisfactorily
delayed through sex education or counseling,
which is quite often the case, sex therapy is necessary. Traditionally, two procedures have been
used to teach males how to slow down their ejaculatory responses. Perhaps the best known of these
is the "squeeze technique" of Masters and Johnson
(1970); the other method is the "start-stop technique" developed by James H. Semans (1956). Both
techniques have several things in common: they
both require that the dysfunctional couple discontinue their usual coital activities until therapy is over; both demand the complete cooperation
of the female partner; both employ sensate focus
sexual pleasuring; both limit genital contact to
that required by the treatment procedures; both
seek to teach ejaculatory control by emphasizing
pre-ejaculatory awareness; and both can be used
in a flexible treatment program that may include
not only ongoing sex education, but also relationship counseling and/or psychotherapy when indicated.

The start-stop technique

Once the couple has discontinued their prescribed activities and reduced their anxieties
through sexual pleasuring, they are ready to
learn ejaculatory control. The start-stop method, also known as the "Semans technique," is
quite simple. It begins with the extravaginal
stimulation of the penis by the female partner.
When this has been sufficiently exciting to
bring the male close to ejaculation, he informs
his partner and she stops masturbating him until
the ejaculatory urge subsides. Then, at his request, the sexual stimulation is resumed. (This

Notes:

Notes:

start-stop exercise should be repeated at least
four times, in close succession, without ejaculation; if the male does ejaculate the series must
be restarted -- after a suitable period of rest.)

After several days of successful control,
the couple is asked to include a lubricant in
their start-stop exercises. This is the logical
next step since ejaculation occurs more quickly
while the penis is wet. When they have been repeatedly successful under these circumstances, "it
can be expected that the moist surface of the vagina will no longer produce premature ejaculation"
(Semans, 1956, p. 354).

Helen Kaplan (1975) then adds a third step
-- intravaginal containment -- to the Semans technique. She recommends that the couple continue to
practice their start-stop exercises during coitus,
first with the woman in the female superior position, and then side to side. This additional
training should increase ejaculatory control and
give each partner a greater sense of confidence.

Using the Semans technique, with Kaplan's
modifications, satisfactory ejaculatory control
should be obtained in three to six weeks. Semans
himself devoted an average of three and a third
office hours to each case (1956); other therapists
may not work this quickly.

The squeeze technique

The squeeze technique of Masters and Johnson
(1970) is very similar to that recommended by
J.H. Semans. Initially, the male reclines and the
female stimulates his penis. Unlike the start-stop
method, however, she performs a "squeeze" (just be-
low the rim of the glans -- see Figure 5, p. 59
when he announces his urge to ejaculate. Once
these feelings have subsided, the masturbation/
squeeze routine should be resumed and repeated
three or four times in close succession without
the male ejaculating.

When these tasks have been accomplished, the
couple is ready for intravaginal containment.
Again, however, instead of just "stopping" when her
partner tells her of his urge to ejaculate, the
woman -- who is in the superior coital position --
removes his penis from her vagina and squeezes it.
Then, after the ejaculatory urge has passed, she
places the penis back inside her vagina and the
routine is repeated two or three more times a day
for several days.

Using the squeeze technique, satisfactory

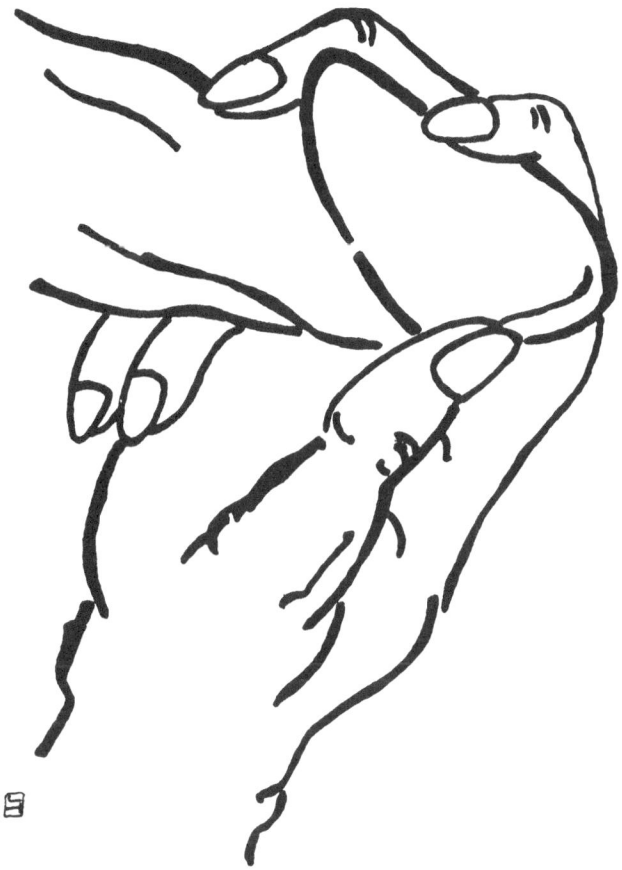

Figure 5: Squeeze Technique

Notes:

ejaculatory control should be obtained in two to six weeks. Levine (1976a) recommends that sex therapists expect to spend from six to ten office sessions with each couple.

Results of Treatment

Helen Kaplan (1975) describes premature ejaculation as "the favorite dysfunction of sex therapists because although it is highly prevalent and troublesome, it is extremely easy to treat with sex therapy in most cases" (p. 152). Her impression as to the "treatability" of premature ejaculation is supported by both Masters and Johnson (1970) and Semans (1956) who report 98% and 100% "cure rates" respectively. This is not to say that there will be no problems incurred during the course of treatment, but, on the average, sex therapists should have little problem treating and delaying premature ejaculation.

Retarded Ejaculation

In retarded ejaculation there is an involuntary overcontrol or inhibition of the ejaculatory reflex. This means that males with this disorder may not evidence any other dysfunctional sexual behavior (e.g., impotence) since only the orgasmic/ejaculatory phase of their sexual response cycle has been affected. In fact, it is often the case that this behavioral inhibition is itself only a partial or selective sexual dysfunction, occurring only under certain circumstances. For example, the patient may note the inability to ejaculate intravaginally (with coitus), but his masturbatory response may not be affected at all. In other cases, however, the symptoms may be more severe with the man being unable even to masturbate to orgasm when a woman is in the room with him. Naturally, there are also instances of very mild symptoms wherein the ejaculation is just profoundly delayed, eventually occurring after lengthy and vigorous coital thrusting.

Diagnosis

Sexual history

A thorough review of the sex therapy literature reveals that most writers in this field believe that retarded ejaculation is almost always a partial, situational, and/or transitory disorder, and that only rarely does the dysfunctional patient note that he has never experienced ejaculation. These secondary characteristics suggest that retarded ejaculation develops as a result of trauma, and that orgastic response

becomes unconsciously restricted to "safe" situations -- such as private masturbation.

In cases of retarded ejaculation, the sex
history should give special attention to those
events or attitudes that may have taught the male
to associate sexual activity and/or genital intimacy with pain or religious disapproval (i.e., "sin,"
as he perceives it), thereby precipitating anxiety
and guilt as involuntary conditioned responses to
sexual stimulation. For example, the therapist
should try to find out if the patient was ever interrupted during sex play and punished. Did he
ever become involved in a premarital pregnancy?
What are his religious views concerning intercourse?
Does he see sex as dirty? What were the early conditioning experiences of his sexual partner?
(Since she probably exerts a considerable influence
on his sexual performance, her views on these and
similar topics must be explored.)

Practical issues may also be involved. How
does the couple feel about pregnancy and parenthood? Is he comfortable with, and confident in,
the contraceptive protection he and his partner are
using?

Answers to these questions, along with other
information that will round-out the couple's sexual
profiles, should give the sex therapist insight into the nature and dynamics of the dysfunctional
symptoms -- disclosing how they affect the interaction between the retarded ejaculator and his sexual partner. Naturally, a differential diagnosis
will still require a medical evaluation and possibly even a psychiatric interview.

Medical evaluation

Organic illness is usually not a factor in
retarded ejaculation (A.M.A., 1972). In fact, some
writers (Kales, Martin, and Franchini, 1977) report
that the only exceptions to the psychogenic origins
of this sexual dysfunction are neurological disorders,
and the ingestion of certain drugs (e.g., Mellaril
and certain antihypertensive medications) which may
adversely affect the ejaculatory response. Helen
Kaplan (1974b) agrees with their assessment, but
she cautions that the sex therapist must be alert
to possible organic involvement "even when the patient's symptoms can readily be explained by his psychosexual history, his marital relationship, etc."
(p. 321). This suggests that, although the possibility of medical problems is slight, a thorough medical evaluation -- including a complete physical examination -- is recommended when working with retarded ejaculation.

Notes:

Psychiatric/psychological evaluation

A multiplicity of factors can bring on retarded ejaculation. Masters and Johnson (1970)
note that conflicts arising from religious orthodoxy are the most common cause, but they add that
the male's fear of pregnancy or his lack of interest in or physical attraction to his partner are
also frequently involved. Therefore, whenever the
sexual history or other materials reveal the
presence of unresolved conflicts (either emotional or interpersonal), anger, fear, or guilt, a
psychiatric/psychological evaluation is recommended.

Diagnostic conclusions

Organic factors will be ruled out, in almost every instance, in favor of a psychogenic
etiology. This being the case, treatment will consist of various (nonmedical)efforts designed to
reverse this specific inhibitory reflex. Sometimes this can be achieved through sex education
and counseling, but frequently sex therapy tech-
nicians are also required.

Treatment: Sex Education and Counseling

Sex education

If sexual ignorance is suspected as the
problem, appropriate education should be directed toward the couple. For example, if the sexual history or the psychiatric evaluation suggests
that the man is inhibiting his ejaculatory reflex
because he fears pregnancy, and that he is neither comfortable with nor confident in the contraceptive methods he and his partner are using, the
most appropriate treatment may consist of simple
contraceptive education and possibly a referral
to the necessary source of supply (physician,
drug store, etc.).

Sexual information examination

Since retarded ejaculation is a sexual dysfunction precipitated most often by the male's
anxieties concerning sexual stimulation via the
female genitalia, a sexological examination is
almost always appropriate. Indeed, any event or
procedure that can dispel ignorance or quiet anxiety can be helpful. Naturally, a general type
of verbal sex education should be carried on with
the couple during this process since it is unlikely that either their ignorance or their anxieties are limited just to sexual anatomy.

Psychotherapy

When the patient's ejaculatory response is inhibited because of intrapsychic or social conflicts, it may be necessary to order psycho-therapeutic intervention. This is often the case when the patient perceives his sexual urges or be-haviors as "sinful" (Masters and Johnson, 1970), and evidences any of the typical symptoms of anx-iety, guilt or anger. In other instances, a path-ological fear of pregnancy and/or parenthood may require psychotherapeutic attention since it is un-likely that the male will be able to ejaculate in-travaginally when such a fear is preoccupying his attention.

Relationship counseling

It is not uncommon for sexual disorders to be either caused or compounded by problems within the relationship. R.W. Taylor (1975) notes one such case wherein retarded ejaculation resulted from the woman's recriminations after her partner's condom burst during intercourse. In this instance, reports Taylor, treatment consisted of establish-ing the point of conflict, and the "cure" resulted from the couple's relational conflicts being re-solved.

Naturally, other similar examples could be of-fered, but the facts seem clear: when the ejacula-tion is inhibited because of relational stress, that stress must be removed before adequate sexual func-tioning can be restored (Zussman and Zussman, 1976). Sometimes this can be accomplished by counseling alone, but frequently relationship counseling will only be a helpful adjunct to other treatment tech-niques (Kales et al., 1977).

Treatment: Sex Therapy

It is likely that sex education and counsel-ing will be very helpful to many couples who evi-dence retarded ejaculation. Frequently, however, those treatment techniques will need to be supple-mented with certain behavioral tasks that can help recondition the inadequate ejaculatory response.

Prohibitions and prescriptions

To interrupt the further reinforcement of the inadequate ejaculatory response, all recre-ational coital activities are prohibited and geni-tal intimacy is restricted to the sexual tasks pre-scribed by the therapist. Non-genital pleasuring is regularly employed to reduce anxiety and create a sense of physical intimacy -- without the threat

Notes:

of sexual/genital inadequacy. (In some cases, where the dysfunctional symptoms are only slight, genital pleasuring may begin at the start of therapy. For most couples, however, genital intimacy should be delayed until the therapist is sure that the male patient is comfortable enough with his partner to allow that degree of physical intimacy.)

Progressive desensitization and directed masturbation

In the beginning of therapy the male is directed to masturbate[1] -- to erotic fantasy -- with his sexual partner as close to him as he can tolerate. (Some men will not be able to ejaculate with her in the same house; others, however, can successfully ejaculate with her outside the bedroom door -- or even closer.) He is then asked to have her move closer to him, as he becomes more comfortable with her presence during subsequent ejaculations. Then, as his anxiety progressively decreases, he will be able to tolerate her manual stimulation of his genitals, and eventually these procedures will culminate in his successful intravaginal ejaculation.

Masters and Johnson (1970) suggest that once the male has successfully ejaculated via his partner's manual stimulation, he is ready for intravaginal ejaculation. They recommend that this step be attempted with the female in the superior position; this will allow her to take responsibility for the demanding pelvic thrusts that are a necessary part of coital stimulation.

If ejaculation is not accomplished in this fashion, they then recommend that all pelvic thrusting cease and that the couple return to the manual stimulation of the penis. Then, with the male announcing that he has reached the point of ejaculatory inevitability, his partner quickly reinserts the penis into her vagina: "It matters not if she is a little too late in her intromission efforts.... Even if but a few drops of ejaculate are accepted intravaginally, the mental bock against intravaginal ejaculation will suffer some

---

[1]Geboes, Omer and DeMoor (1975) recommend the use of an electric vibrator with those men who have trouble ejaculating under such circumstances: "The electrical current of this apparatus causes vibrations in the tip of the instrument and thus highly stimulates the glans penis when the tip is brought into contact during erection. Ejaculation and orgasm may follow after 3 to 6 minutes" (p. 1019).

cracks" (Masters and Johnson, 1970, p.131).   Notes:

Procedural variations

Helen Kaplan (1974b): 1975) follows an almost identical treatment plan with re arded ejacu-
lators but she differs from Masters and Johnson by
recommending that vaginal penetration and ejaculation occur with the male entering from either the
superior position, or from behind ("doggy fashion"),
so that his partner can offer him added genital stimulation. Zussman and Zussman suggest that an in-
termediate step -- between manual stimulation and
vaginal penetration -- may be necessary. Specifically, they recommend (1976) that once the male has
ejaculated in the presence of his sexual partner,
he may then need to learn to ejaculate near her vagina (or on it) before he will be able to accomplish
intravaginal emission.

Results of Treatment

Using the treatment techniques and procedures
outlined above, retarded ejaculation can be effectively treated.[1] Naturally, the therapist must be prepared to meet some resistance even among the most co-
operative couples and sometimes an angry spouse will
deliberately sabotage the treatment program, but
dramatic delays or failures are the exception. Most
often therapy progresses according to plan, and the
couple experiences success in a relatively short
period of time. In fact, as Helen Kaplan (1974b)
has pointed out, "patients whose inhibited ejaculations are relatively independent of deeper psychopathology seem to have an excellent prognosis with
sex therapy" (p. 336).

FEMALE SEXUAL DYSFUNCTIONS

Orgastic Dysfunction

The fact that many women in our culture are
unable to achieve orgasm/climax has made <u>anorgasmia</u>

---

[1]Masters and Johnson (1970) do not speak in
terms of "cure," but they note only three instances of failure among the seventeen patients
(17.6%) they treated. This implies a success rate
of 82.4%, which is better than that of Geboes et
al. (1975), who succeeded with 72% of their patients. Helen Kaplan (1974b) also speaks optimis-
tically, but she modestly reports that her own
"experience thus far has been too limited to be
statistically significant" (p. 336).

Notes:

the classical female sexual disorder in America.[1] As with other types of sexual nonresponsiveness, an orgastic dysfunction can be designated either primary (having never occurred under any circumstances) or secondary (developing after a period of adequate orgasmic response).

A diagnosis of primary orgastic dysfunction is indicated when the patient reports that she has never experienced orgasm. (These symptoms are usually designated preorgasmia -- a term which reflects the belief that all women are potentially orgastic.) Secondary anorgasmia, on the other hand, is a term which indicates that the orgastic inhibition has developed after a period of adequate sexual functioning. A secondary orgastic inhibition may be either complete or situational. When it is complete, the women no longer experiences orgasm under any circumstances; when it is situational, however, she may be orgastic with direct manual or oral clitoral stimulation but not with coitus or vice versa, or she may periodically lose the ability to climax from any type of erotic stimulation.

Diagnosis

Sexual history

Aside from the medical evaluation, the sexual history is the most important clinical tool available for discovering the origins of orgastic problems. As with all other sexual disorders, the therapist should attempt to identify the nature and duration of the dysfunctional symptoms and the degree of residual sexual response remaining. That is to say, is the disorder of a primary or secondary nature? If it is secondary, how and under what circumstances did it first occur? Is it constant or episodic; situational, selective or general; and to what degree is the patient able to enjoy coitus?[2]

----

[1]Kinsey (1953) reported that 10 - 15% of married women in America have never experienced orgasm. This figure was confirmed again in 1973 by Hunt, who undertook a survey sponsored by the Playboy Foundation.

[2]It is important to note that some women do not find orgasm particularly important, or at least for some it is not an essential part of every coital experience. In these cases, therapy should only be initiated when the woman feels that she is missing something, or when she wants to change either the circumstances under which she is now orgastic or

When the patient admits to preorgasmia, the therapist should explore her understanding of, and feelings about, human sexuality; it may be that she has simply never learned to climax. This is often the case when the woman has negative feelings about her own genitalia which have prevented her from exploring her own sexual anatomy and practicing orgastic response through masturbation.[1]

When the patient describes secondary symptoms, however, the therapist must expand the clinical perspective to include information about her sexual partner and their relationship. For instance, it may be that he is not spending enough time or providing adequate sexual stimulation for her to be orgastically responsive during coitus; after all, he could be an undiagnosed premature ejaculator. On the other hand, she may be quite angry with him, or no longer love him, and her orgasmic inhibition is her way of expressing these negative feelings.

Once these developmental/social factors have been covered and an accurate profile of the dysfunctional patient has been established (her partner) must be included in this evaluation when the sexual history indicates secondary symptoms), she should then undergo a comprehensive medical evaluation to determine -- or rule out -- organic pathology and/or anatomical problems that may be inhibiting her orgastic response.

Medical evaluation

Anorgasmia is usually psychogenic in origin, but it is vital that each patient undergo a thorough pelvic examination to assure that there are no organic or anatomical problems that could prevent her from experiencing sexual arousal or inhibit her response to that stimulation. For example, when examining a preorgastic woman, the physician must establish that she possesses a sexually functional pelvic anatomy and that her inhibited sexual response is not a symptom of vaginal or clitoral abnormalities, pelvic disease, or chronic infection (e.g., vaginal trichomoniasis or mycosis). In the case of secondary nonorgasmia, the examiner must not only check the patient for organic disease and/or chronic infection, but the possibility of v inal trauma

Notes:

---

[1] Masters and Johnson (1966) report that 94.5% of the women who never masturbated remain preorgasmic. Colgan (1977) elaborates on this issue: "Clearly, if a woman has never masturbated because she is disgusted by the idea, she will also have difficulty enjoying sex in coitus. And if she has negative feelings about her own body, she will have difficulty sharing it freely and lovingly with someone else" (p. 10).

Notes: e.g., rape, surgery, childbirth, etc.) must also
                      be considered.[1]

                          Psychiatric psychological evaluation

                          Traditionally, psychiatric literature
                      (Fenichel, 1945; Freud, 1959, etc.) has equated
                      anorgasmia with psychopathology; but correct find-
                      ings tend to challenge that view.[2]

                          This changing attitude among clinicians
                      and theorists, however, should not suggest that
                      anorgastic women are necessarily free from, or
                      that their sexual responses have not been ad-
                      versely affected by, various intrapsychic or rela-
                      tional conflicts -- for this is certainly not al-
                      ways the case. As a matter of fact, Kaplan (1974b)
                      nas noted that orgastic response can be easily con-
                      ditioned, and that once this response pattern has
                      been inhibited (e.g., due to guilt, depression,
                      etc.) it continues in that manner almost automati-

---

[1]When the secondary symptoms are situational
in nature, the physician should suspect that while
the patient's vaginal anatomy is "normal," it may
not permit her to experience adequate sexual a-
rousal in certain circumstances (e.g., coitus) because of its own unique structure. These conditions
(e.g., a large or very heavy clitoral hood) may or
may not requre medical/surgical attention (Crist,
1977; Isenberg and Elting, 1976), but it is important that they be diagnoised and that the patient, her sexual partner, and the sex therapist be
aware of them so that their affects may be taken
into account (Huffman, 1976).

[2]For instance, Munjack and Staples (1976)
report that while it is true that some studies
have discovered a correlation between such personality traits as hostility (Cooper, 1969),
dominance (DeMartino, 1963), neuroticism
(Eysenck, 1971), neurasthenia (Terman, 1938),
and certain types of sexual functioning, others
(Fisher and Osofsky, 1967; Freedman, 1965;
Kleegman, 1959, Landis, Bolles and D'Esopo, 1940;
Miller and Wilson, 1968; Uddenberg, 1974; Winokur,
1963; Winokur and Gaston, 1961; and Winokur and
Holeman, 1963) have found little or no connection.
As a matter of fact, with the possible exclusion
of mania (Allison and Wilson, 1960; Cassidy et al.,
1957), depression (Winokur, 1963), hysteria
(Purtell, Robins and Cohn, 1954), and organic
brain syndrome (Winokur, 1963), there seem to be
no clear or consistent connections between psychiatric diagnosis and adequate sexual response
(Munjack and Staples, 1976).

cally. Therefore, with some patients, under certain circumstances, a psychiatric evaluation may be the appropriate diagnostic tool to aid the sex therapist in establishing, or ruling out, the existence of significant psychological/social factors in the etiology of the orgastic dysfunction. Most often, however, this will not be necessary since the dynamics of the sexual inhibition should become readily apparent in the taking of the sexual history.

Diagnostic conclusions

Usually orgastic dysfunction is emotionally based, with sexual ignorance, anxiety, and relational factors being important contributing factors. This means that, in most cases, both sex education and counseling will be the appropriate first steps in treatment -- with sex therapy being reserved for those more difficult cases where the orgasmic response remains firmly inhibited, or where it is due to severe intrapsychic or social conflicts.

Treatment: Sex Education and Counseling

Sex education

Preorgasmia is often the result of sexual anxiety, ignorance and/or poor sexual technique. Sometimes the preorgastic woman is completely unaware of her own genital structure -- having never examined herself "down there." (This view is easily fostered by parents who scold their children for touching their genitals: "Don't do that -- now go wash your hands!") In other instances the patient's religious or ethical views may have kept her from experimenting with masturbation, or with other stimulating techniques that might have brought on an orgastic response.

In these cases, as with most preorgastic women, an important first step in treatment is sex education. They should be taught that their genitalia need not be dirty, that sexual pleasure is good, and that it is all right for them to actively pursue their own sexual gratification. They must also learn about sexual anatomy, sexual psychophysiology, and sexual technique. Then masturbation training can begin.

Self-stimulation is an essential part of treatment. The patient must first learn how to stimulate herself to climax before she can teach this to her sexual partner. Moreover, the privacy of this solitary act will allow her time to practice and she can become orgastic on her own schedule -- unpressured. (An electric vibrator may be helpful in some cases.)

Notes:

After the patient has been repeatedly successful experiencing orgasm in this way, she can attempt coitus. Often, **the transference of orgasm from**
masturbation to coitus will not be difficult, but
if it is, the sex therapist may schedule to see both
partners together to insure that appropriate coital
technique and adequate sexual (clitoral) stimulation are being offered. When this problem persists
the woman is then considered to have secondary situational symptoms, and treatment should shift its
focus to include the couple.

Sexual information examination

The preorgasmic woman may have a very poor or
inaccurate understanding of sexual anatomy. A sexological examination of her own genitalia, along
with instructions on self-stimulation techniques,
can greatly assist in her treatment program.

In cases of secondary anorgasmia the sexological examination may not be necessary since the
secondary nature of the dysfunction indicates that
the sexual inhibition is a reaction to something.
Nevertheless, if the sex therapist feels that it
might be helpful, the sexological examination of
both partners should be included. This is especially true when the woman is suffering from situational
anorgasmia; that is, when she is easily orgasmic
with masturbation or with other sexual partners. In
this situation it could be that her current partner
is the one needing the sex education.

Psychotherapy

Psychopathology is usually not a factor in
anorgasmia. Despite this, however, the sex therapist
must be alert to situational, or transient, affective disorders (e.g., anxiety, depression, guilt,
etc.) that may be playing a part in the etiology of
the sexual dysfunction. When these do occur they
can often be effectively treated by medication
(Renshaw, 1975) and/or individual psychotherapy.

Relationship counseling

Secondary anorgasmia is sometimes indicative
of a deteriorating relationship, or of profound
anger between the sexual **partners.** When this is the
case, relationship therapy may assist the couple in
identifying and articulating their problems (Krohne,
1977) and in negotiating an appropriate solution.

Treatment: Sex Therapy

Preorgasmia seems to respond quite well to sex
education and counseling techniques (e.g., Barbach,

1975; Kohlenberg, 1974; LoPiccolo and Lobitz, 1972; **Schneidman and McGuire, 1956; Snyder, LoPiccolo and LoPiccolo, 1975;** Sotile, Kilmann and Follingstad, 1977; etc.), but secondary anorgasmia often requires more direct attention. (For example, after a preorgastic female has learned to respond to self-stimulation, she may still be unable to achieve orgasm through coitus: or in another situation, a woman may remain situationally dysfunctional even though her marital problems have significantly diminished, etc.) Therefore, when treating patients with secondary symptoms the therapist may find that various sex therapy techniques will prove to be helpful adjuncts to the educational/counseling procedures already outlined.

Prohibitions and prescriptions

The usual steps are undertaken: the couple's commitment to sex therapy is explored and articulated; they then agree to postpone all recreational coital contact, and their promises to practice all homework assignments are noted.

Directed masturbation

When the secondary orgastic inhibition is complete, the technique for restoring it is the same as with preorgasmia: directed masturbation. Once orgasm has been achieved in this manner, the patient is encouraged to attempt it via her partner's stimulation.

Sensate focus exercise

If either partner is particularly anxious, the non-genital pleasuring exercises can precede the genital stimulation. Frequently, however, this will not be necessary, and the couple can begin immediately with a sexually stimulating genital caress.

Non-coital orgasm

The woman's first orgasm with her partner should be attempted by non-coital (manual, oral, or mechanical) clitoral stimulation.[1] Coital stimulation will follow after she is very comfortable with her partner's erotic attentions and responds easily to them.

---

[1]Pelvic thrusting is often too clumsy for these initial experiences; therefore, coitus is prohibited during the early part of therapy so

Notes:

Coital orgasm

For some women orgasm via coitus will follow naturally from this "push offered in the previous exercise. If this does not occur, however, extra stimulation may be required; this can be obtained through the "bridge maneuver."

Bridge maneuver

The bridge maneuver is a technique whereby one of the partners directly stimulates the clitoris manually during intercourse (see Figure 6, p. 72). This provides the clitoral stimulation necessary for orgasm that may be too difficult for some women to obtain through intercourse. Once orgasm is achieved in this manner, the couple may be able to modify their sexual technique (positions, duration of intercourse, etc.) so that the bridge is not necessary; but in certain anatomical circumstances this type of extra stimulation may always be necessary.

Results of Treatment

The duration of treatment for anorgasmia

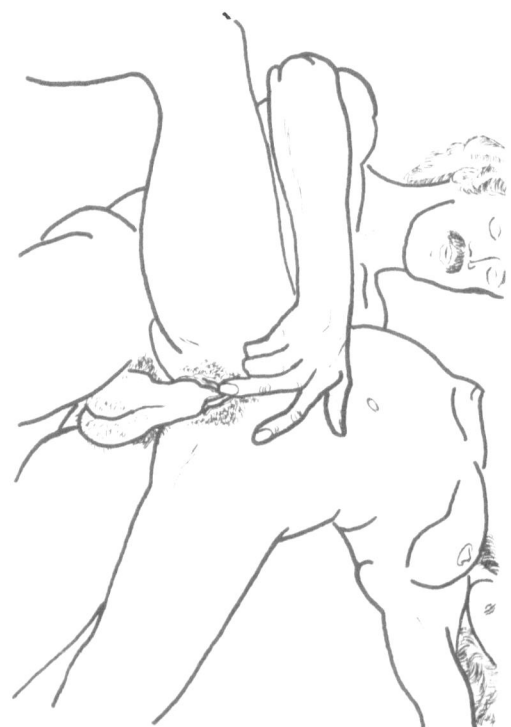

Figure 6:   Bridge Maneuver

differs greatly between therapists. For instance, Blakeney et al., (1976) report good results with a two and a half day workshop approach. Masters and Johnson (1970), on the other hand, devote two full weeks to treatment; while others, like Barbach (1975), are successful in just fifteen hours (spread over a five-week period). Despite these variations, however, all of the sex therapy literature is in agreement on one issue: anorgasmia is a sexual dysfunction that is highly treatable in a a short-term clinical framework using a combination of education, counseling, and behavioral techniques.

Dyspareunia

Dyspareunia is the clinical term for intercourse that is so painful that it interrupts the woman's sexual response cycle during the excitement phase, preventing her from naturally progressing onto plateau and orgasm, and inhibiting her enjoyment of the sex act.[1] This coital discomfort may be due to either emotional or organic factors and it may present itself as either a primary or secondary sexual dysfunction.

Diagnosis

Sexual history

Once the primary or secondary nature of the symptoms has been noted, the therapist should attempt to identify the circumstances under which they occur. For instance if the symptoms are primary, have they occurred with more than one partner? In which positions? Is there adequate foreplay to produce sufficient vaginal lubrication?

With secondary symptoms the sex therapist should explore the possibility of recent physical trauma (e.g., childbirth, surgery, rape, etc.) as well as delving into emotional issues and the couple's relationship. For example, episiotomy scars and changes in the size of the vagina following hysterectomy commonly result in coital pain. On the other hand, a woman's anger toward her husband, or her guilt over a recent affair might result in an affective reaction that could inhibit her vaginal lubrication, resulting in dyspareunia.

---

[1] In dyspareunia, the woman's sexual response cycle is interrupted by coital pain; when sexual stimulation occurs by other methods, such as masturbation, however, her response cycle is not affected -- because there is no accompanying pain -- and orgasm occurs naturally.

Notes:

When the dyspareunia has occurred with only one
partner, the sex therapist must consider the possibility that it may be the male's sexual technique
(i.e., preference for certain positions, desire for
deep vaginal penetration, etc.) that is causing the
coital discomfort. In these situations both mem-
bers of the sexual relationship must be included in
the history-taking and in the treatment program.

Medical evaluation

Due to the fact that medical problems (e.g.,
sensitivity reactions to contraceptive creams, jel-
lies, suppositories, foams, foam tablets, and latex
condoms or diaphrams), organic disease (e.g., vulvovaginitis, endometriosis, pelvic infections, tumors,
cysts, or cancer, etc.), and anatomical or surgical
conditions (e.g., an intact hymen or irritated rem-
nants of hymen, perineal damage from episiotomies,
colporrhaphy scars, etc.) may very well be involved
in dyspareunia, a complete physical evaluation -- including a thorough pelvic examination -- is necessary with each patient.

Psychiatric/psychological evaluation

Psychopathology is usually not a factor in the
etiology of dyspareunia (Munjack and Staples, 1976).
Nevertheless, the sex therapist may choose to order
a psychiatric consultation, along with a screening
M.M.P.I., as part of the patient's diagnostic profile. Most often this will indicate the presence of
only minor, transient, situational disturbances; occasionally, however, a comprehensive mental status
evaluation will show that the dysfunctional symptoms
are actually the patient's reaction to a profound
fear of penetration (e.g., following rape, or due to
fears of an unwanted pregnancy, etc.) that might, if
left untreated, develop into severe vaginismus.

Diagnostic conclusions

Frequently, if not most often, the causes of
dyspareunia are physical rather than psychological.
Connell (1975, p. 61) implies that this is fortunate
because "the physical causes of dyspareunia, either
congenital or acquired, are relatively easy to diag-
nose and treat."

Sometimes, however, dyspareunia can have a
psychogenic basis. When this is the case the coital
pain is usually due to insufficient vaginal lubricatic
(This inadequate sexual response -- which is caused
by an interruption of the excitement phase of the
woman's sexual response cycle -- can occur for a
variety of reasons: insufficient foreplay, an inability to think or feel sexually, anxiety about sexual

performance, assuming a spectator role during coitus, fear of pain and/or pregnancy, fear of social compromise, lesbian orientation, etc.) Patients with symptoms of this type often respond well to sex education and counseling.[1]

Treatment: Sex Education And Counseling

Sex education

Sexual ignorance is often a precipitating factor in dyspareunia. For instance, when the coital pain is due to the vagina being too dry (which is common in psychogenic dyspareunia), it may be that the couple does not have an adequate understanding of sexual psychophysiology and they are attempting penile penetration too soon. This problem usually responds well to an improvement in arousal (foreplay) technique, which means that the sex therapists may need to discuss such things as genital petting and oral sex. (The therapist's "permission" to undertake these activities can be a very important element in treatment.)

In other cases, painful intercourse may be the result of poor coital technique (e.g., awkward positions, restricted movements, or deep vaginal thrusting, etc.) that can be easily corrected. Often, just a simple change in position can make a great difference in the sexual experience. (Again, the therapist's "permission" to experiment can be powerful "medicine.")

Sexual information examination

The sexological examination can be very helpful in treating dyspareunia. For example, when inadequate vaginal lubrication is the problem, both partners should be shown how the vagina reacts to sexual stimulation, and how lubrication occurs. Likewise, when the problem is based in the man's desire to thrust deeply -- perhaps causing the penis to bump into the cervix -- he can be shown that the vagina is not an "endless pit," and he can then understand that plunging deeply into the vagina can hurt his partner. (It may also help to point out that his erect penis is of "normal" size; some men are concerned about such things, and this type of comment can be reassuring. Never miss an opportunity to reduce anxiety!)

---

[1]Lesbians who marry males for socioeconomic reasons have a less favorable prognosis.

Notes:

Psychotherapy

When the sexual history or the psychiatric
evaluation suggests that the woman's excitement
phase is being interrupted (i.e., the mechanisms
leading to vaginal lubrication are being inhibited)
because of intrapsychic conflicts (e.g., anxiety,
guilt, depression, etc.), psychotherapy is recommended. Sex education, however, may still be an
important aspect of this phase of treatment.

Relationship counseling

When the sexual inhibition is due to conflict
within, or a deterioration of, the patient's relationship, therapy focusing on their interaction
(marriage counseling) may be the treatment of
choice. Indeed, it could be that anger, mistrust,
and/or fear has infiltrated and destroyed the couple's former sense of intimacy and the coital discomfort is a secondary symptom.[1] In such cases conjoint therapy -- sometimes including sex education
-- can be very helpful.

Treatment: Sex Therapy

When sex education and counseling, by themselves, have not been sufficient to reverse the sexual inhibition that has brought on the dispareunia,
it may be necessary to incorporate the sensate focus
pleasuring techniques in the treatment plan.

Prohibitions and prescriptions

Naturally, the usual precautions are observed:
once the couple has noted their commitment to therapy, they must then agree to postpone all recreational coital contact and promise to practice their
homework assignments as directed.

Non-genital pleasuring

When extremes in affect are a factor, the
sensate focus should begin with non-genital pleasuring. This approach can be particularly helpful
as an adjunct to relationship therapy; it often
helps the couple to renew their sense of physical

-----

[1]Spano and Lamont (1975) note that both con-
scious and unconscious expressions of relational
problems are common causes of dyspareunia: "Issues
of control figure largely in such situations. A
woman may feel that the sexual relationship is the
only domain within the partnership that she can control" (p. 24).

intimacy without (prematurely) involving them in
sexual contact.

Genital pleasuring

Once both partners are comfortable with non-
genital pleasuring, they can begin the sexually
arousing erotic techniques that are part of the
genital message. (This is also a good opportunity for them to experiment with oral sex, if they
choose, since that may be a very effective way
to bring on vaginal lubrication.)

Coitus

Sexual intercourse can resume once the vaginal lubrication is sufficient to permit comfortable penile penetration.

Results Of Treatment

Those problems that require medical attention are usually treated quickly and show good
results. Psychogenic dyspareunia also responds
well to the sex therapy approaches described but
the duration of treatment may be somewhat longer,
depending on the problems encountered and the
depth of therapy required for symptom relief.
Ideally, however, the couple should experience
substantial improvement within two to five weeks.

Vaginismus

Vaginismus is an involuntary spasm -- or
conditioned response -- of the pubococcygeus
muscle which makes vaginal penetration very difficult or impossible. This psychosomatic reaction may be emotionally based or there may be
some organic involvement (e.g., vaginitis, pelvic inflammatory disease, etc.). Usually, however, its etiology is solely psychogenic.

This excitement phase disorder may present
itself as either a primary or secondary sexual
dysfunction. In primary vaginismus the problem-
atic muscular conditioning appears to have always existed and vaginal penetration of any type
has never been possible, even by a tampon or during a pelvic examination by a physician. Secondary vaginismus, on the other hand, indicates a
conditioned response of the pubococcygeus muscle-
group which has developed after a period of adequate sexual functioning. In almost all cases
this conditioning is complete or total, and the
dysfunctional behavior does not occur just situationally or episodically.

Notes:

Diagnosis

Sexual history

After outlining the nature of the sexual
symptoms, the therapist should attempt a brief developmental profile of the vaginismic patient.
For instance, a young woman who was reared in an
atmosphere of strong religious orthodoxy may not
feel free to indulge herself in an activity that
is so self-gratifying; moreover, the punitive
nature of her upbringing ("Thou shalt not!") may
also prevent her from relaxing and enjoying this
erotic act (Noonan, 1966). This early conditioning, in fact, may have trained her to exclude sexual activities from her list of "acceptable" be-
haviors. (Vaginismus is a very "protective,"
self-serving symptom for these individuals; it
keeps them from being able to submit to those
carnal desires which they have been taught to
find so objectionable.)

Naturally, secondary symptoms may indicate
the need to include the sexual partner in the
diagnostic/treatment format. For example, vaginismus may be the woman's way of responding to her
partner's premature ejaculation ("I won't let him
disappoint me again") or it may indicate that she
is insecure in the relationship and that she does
not want him that close. On the other hand, if
she has a strong homosexual orientation, she
might find sex with a male partner particularly
offensive; the vaginismic response may be her way
of expressing this distaste.

Medical evaluation

A thorough pelvic examination of the vaginismic partner is essential for two reasons. First,
vaginismus may be the result of organically based,
chronic dyspareunia that will require medical attention; second, once all organic factors have
been ruled out, the pelvic examination may be helpful in demonstrating to the patient the psychosomatic basis of the disorder. (This latter point is
especially true with primary symptoms wherein all
vaginal penetration is prevented.)

Psychiatric/psychological evaluation

A psychiatric consultation may be particularly helpful when working with patients who evidence primary symptoms. This is because, in primary vaginismus, the conditioned response is not
limited to sexual penetration -- suggesting that a
more pervasive emotional pathology may be involved.

Diagnostic conclusions

Vaginismus is almost always psychogenic, but it may occasionally be secondary to chronic dyspareunia wherein organic factors have played some part. Naturally, if physical problems are present, they must be treated medically; usually, however, both primary and secondary vaginismus are the direct result of anxiety (e.g., a fear of penetration, physical pain, abandonment, etc.) and its treatment is best approached through educational/psychotherapeutic, and/or behavioral sex therapy techniques.

Treatment: Sex Education and Counseling

Sex education

An educational approach to vaginismus is very effective with secondary symptoms. This is especially true when the vaginismic response is an extreme symptom of chronic, psychogenic dyspareunia. In these cases, inadequate foreplay, poor sexual technique, and/or inaccurate sexual information may have precipitated the coital pain which eventually escalated into a vaginismic spasm. Sex education, within this context, would include all of those measures already outlined in the previous section dealing with dyspareunia additionally, however, this educational approach also emphasizes the positive factors that comprise a healthy sexual relationship (e.g., intimacy, companionship, and love, etc.) in an effort to further combat both anxiety and guilt.

Sexual information examination

The sexological examination can be just as effective in treating vaginismus as it is with dyspareunia. Indeed, as Zussman and Zussman (1976) point out, once the couple sees the involuntary muscular response, they are in a much better position to understand their sexual disorder and to reverse its symptoms:

> A physical examination with both partners ...present is of extreme importance in a case of vaginismus. The mere demonstration to the couple of the spasm of the vaginal muscle helps to focus the problem and prepares them to start immediate therapy. Often the couple is unaware before this demonstration of what is physically causing the barrier to penetration. [p. 124].

Occasionally, this more thorough under-

Notes:

standing combined with sex education is enough to reverse the vaginismic response. More frequently, however, both counseling and sex therapy will still be necessary.

Psychotherapy

In addition to the conditioned response that involuntarily closes the vaginal opening, most vaginismic women are also phobic of intercourse. (This is certainly understandable since coitus has become a physically painful and emotionally uncomfortable activity for them.) Therefore, it is often necessary to confront this additional problem through psychotherapy. Sometimes, however, these feelings cannot be entirely worked through in individual counseling and conjoint sessions are necessary. This is particularly true when there is significant anger in or a profound deterioration of the couple's relationship.

Relationship counseling

As with dyspareunia, relational problems can also be a factor in vaginismus. In effect, the vaginal spasm is the woman's unconscious attempt at "closing him out." In actuality, this may be exactly what she feels she would like to do (exclude him from an intimate relationship), but for some reason she has not. Once these feelings have been articulated, however, and her partner has become aware of the dynamic interplay between her feelings, the relationship, and the sexual dysfunction, resolution of the conflict (and the vaginismic symptom) is possible.

Treatment: Sex Therapy

When sex education and counseling have not been able to satisfactorily reverse the conditioned vaginal response, behavioral sex therapy techniques may be helpful.

Prohibitions and prescriptions

As usual, the couple is asked to discontinue their recreational sexual activities and to practice their homework assignments as prescribed.

Dilatation

The goal of treatment is to cause the extinction of the previously noted vaginal conditioning. This is best accomplished by desensitizing the spastic vaginal inlet through the introduction of objects -- gradually increasing in

size[1] -- into the vaginal entrance. Kaplan (1975)
notes that when the patient can tolerate a phal-
lus-size object, she is cured.

Self-dilatation

This procedure begins with the woman dila-
tating herself vaginally with gradually increasing dilators. Once she is comfortable containing a penis size dilator, she is asked to include her partner in these tasks.

Dilatation by partner

At her request the male then repeats this
procedure. Eventually he is asked to replace the
vaginal dilators with his fingers -- first one
by itself, then two together. As he slowly
moves these in and out of her vagina, she accus-
toms herself to having him inside her.

Sensate focus pleasuring

These vaginal dilatation exercises are also accompanied by both the non-genital and the
genital pleasuring massages. These aid in the
reduction of anxiety and they also contribute to
the couple's feelings of physical intimacy.

Penile penetration

When the female partner is ready, penile
penetration can be attempted. This is done very
slowly, under her guidance, and without coital
thrusting. (The object is to allow her to become comfortable with penile containment.) Then,
at her request, he withdraws.

Coitus

Penile penetration should be repeated several times until the female partner is very comfortable containing an erect penis. Then, when
she is prepared for more activity, regular coitus is permitted.

Results Of Treatment

Depending on the individuals involved and

---

[1]Some therapists recommend the use of grad-
uated rubber or glass catheters for this purpose.
Another technique is to ask the patient to pur-
chase a variety of candles -- starting out with
birthday candles and then larger ones. This is
a distinct advantage because the patients can
take these home with them.

Notes:

Notes:

their relationship, desensitization to the point of cure can be a relatively quick and easy procedure. Kaplan (1975) reflects this optimism when she states: "The positive outcome of treatment by deconditioning the spastic vaginal response is virtually universal providing the couple completes the course of treatment" (p. 110). On the other hand, when extreme interpersonal or relational conflicts accompany the dysfunctional behavior, treatment may take somewhat longer. Despite this variation in the duration of treatment, however, good results are to be expected.[1]

General Sexual Dysfunction

General sexual dysfunction is described by Kaplan (1974b) as the most severe of the female inhibitions. Women suffering from this excitement phase disorder derive little or no pleasure from sexual activity, and they frequently do not respond to sexual stimulation with vaginal lubrication[2], even though they may be orgastic with masturbation.

General sexual dysfunction may present itself either as a primary or secondary sexual disorder, and the secondary symptoms may be isolated to particular situations or partners.

Diagnosis

Sexual history

After noting the primary or secondary nature of the dysfunctional symptoms, the sex therapist should attempt to profile the woman's sexual development and ascertain the condition of the relationship she has with her sexual partner. If

---

[1]Masters and Johnson (1970) report 100% cure in their 29 cases. Kaplan (1974b) notes that 100% of the patients can be cured by combined desensitization and dilatation with psychotherapeutic intervention when necessary. Ellison (1968 and 1972) reports approximately 90% cure rate in methods that combine physical examination with psychotherapy. Finally, Fuchs, et al. (1973 and 1975) report 6 of 9 successes by the in vitro technique and 31 of 34 by the in vivo technique (cf. Fertel, 1977).

[2]When intercourse is attempted under these circumstances, dyspareunia results and the disorder is perpetuated.

the disorder is secondary, her partner must also be included in the history-taking/treatment program; when the condition is primary, however, the focus of both the evaluation and treatment is on the dysfunctional individual. In both instances, thorough medical and psychiatric evaluation will be necessary.

Medical evaluation

General sexual dysfunction is a psychogenic disorder, but it may be associated with organic/physical problems. For example, vaginal infections or pelvic disease may have precipitated severe physical pain which caused the woman extreme discomfort during intercourse. Realizing the cause of her pain, she then trained herself to avoid all further experiences of sexual excitement. This type of reaction being a very real possibility in all cases of general sexual inhibition, a comprehensive physical evaluation -- including a thorough pelvic examination -- is a necessary diagnostic tool.

Psychiatric/psychological evaluation

Women suffering with this profound sexual inhibition may have severe interpsychic conflicts associated with sexual activity. (Note that their symptoms prevent them from being "victimized" by their own sexual desires.) Theoretically, for example, some of them may be very religious women who feel that sex is only for procreation and not for recreation. Others may possess very poor self-images, making them feel unworthy of a man's romantic (erotic) attentions, and/or undeserving of sexual pleasure. Occasionally this disorder may also be found to characterize a woman's feelings of dislike for men in general, or for one man in particular; it may also occur in women with homosexual orientations who are repulsed by heterosexual activities.

Therefore, since the mental mechanisms involved in this disorder are quite complex, a comprehensive mental status evaluation -- including both a psychiatric consultation and psychological testing -- is often employed by sex therapists to aid them in developing an accurate diagnostic profile and in creating an appropriate course of treatment.

Diagnostic conclusions

Once all medical complications have been ruled out, which is usually the case, the psychogenic basis of the sexual inhibition is firmly

Notes:

Notes:

established. If, however, it can be demonstrated
that an underlying sexual disorder (e.g. dyspareunia, vaginismus, or even orgastic dysfunction)
has precipated the current problem, steps must be
taken to reverse that disorder. On the other hand,
it may be that severe intrapsychic conflicts or
relational problems are at fault; in such cases,
intensive psychotherapy and/or relationship counseling will be necessary.

Very often, however, these other factors will
not be found to be either precipitating or compli-
cating the general sexual inhibition (or at least
they will not be involved to the point where they
require direct treatment) and the educational/coun-
seling aspects of treatment can be by-passed, making it possible to begin sex therapy at once. (At
other times when counseling of one type or another
is required, it can be carried on concurrently
with the behavioral sex therapy procedures.)

Treatment: Sex Therapy

Helen Kaplan has been the major contributor
to the literature on general sexual nonresponsiveness (1979). She notes (1975) that the basic
treatment approach for this sexual dysfunction is to
structure the woman's subsequent sexual situations so
that she will be able to experience erotic stimuli
while relaxed and secure. In these circumstances
she will be able to positively sensitize herself
to pleasurable sexual experiences and feelings.

Prohibitions and prescriptions

The couple enters this phase of treatment together. (The woman may also be involved in individual psychotherapy.) They are asked to forego all
recreational coital activities and to devote themselves to the tasks outlined for them.

Non-genital pleasuring

If there is a particularly high level of anxiety, the couple is asked to limit the sensate focus massage to the hands. Later, as the woman becomes more comfortable receiving physical pleasure,
the full nude body caress can take place.

Genital pleasuring

As the woman's ability to tolerate physical
intimacy increases, the focus of the exercise
shifts to erotic pleasure. This is done by encour-
aging the couple to focus their attentions on each
other's genitalia, and to incorporate sexually stimulating caresses into their massage technique.

(Occasionally, the sensate focus exercises will
be the object of resistance by the dysfunctional
partner; when and if this occurs, it should be
dealt with in psychotherapy.)

Nondemand coitus

Once the male has obtained a good erection
the woman mounts in the superior position --
maintaining full control of the situation. After
she has become comfortable with the phallus being
in her vagina, she should begin to slowly move up
and down, concentrating on those vaginal sensa-
tions she previously ignored. This exercise
should be continued until she is tired, and repeated daily.

Coitus

Recreational coitus can resume as soon as
the woman feels the desire to do so; but this
should not be rushed. Normally this treatment
program will continue for several weeks before
coital pleasure is present. (Naturally, her
psychotherapy, or their relationship counseling,
may go on longer than that, even after coital
pleasure has been repeated and acknowledged.)

Results Of Treatment

This treatment program, which was developed
at the Cornell Sex Therapy Clinic and outlined
by Helen Kaplan (1974b, 1975), seems to offer a
marked improvement to those "unresponsive women
whose unresponsiveness is caused by immediate
obstacles" (1974b, p. 373). Unfortunately, however, the present state of the art of sex therapy is such that unresponsive women who are
"blocked by deep hostility or conflicts...are
not helped by these brief, experientially oriented methods" (1974b, p. 373). In these cases,
long-term psychotherapy is often the only other
treatment approach available.

CHAPTER 7

Concluding Therapy

The clinical procedures and therapy techniques described in chapter six are the basis
for the new, brief approaches to the diagnosis
and treatment of psychogenic sexual dysfunctions.
Generally speaking, a couple enters sex therapy
because some sexual problem is preventing them
from enjoying their erotic interaction. The
scope of the resulting treatment is usually restricted to the sexual inadequacy itself, and
therapy concludes when the dysfunctional symptoms
have been dramatically modified or completely re-
versed.

BRIEF TREATMENT

Patient Satisfaction

Once the couple acknowledges their satisfaction with having obtained realistic goals,
the regular therapy sessions can be scheduled
less frequently. (Two 50-minute sessions per
week is not uncommon during the beginning of
treatment; after some initial success has been
noted, however, the couple might be given permission to meet with the therapist only once a
week, or once every other week.) Termination
occurs later, with the mutual consent of all concerned.

Consistent Sexual Response

Most often the criteria for discontinuing
therapy are the reversal of the sexual inhibition
and the consistent appearance of complete sexual
response cycles in both partners. Sometimes
this will happen quickly; in such cases, treatment
may be concluded after only a few sessions. At
other times, however, various complications or

Notes:

interruptions can slow down the patient's progress, and extended care will be required.

EXTENDED TREATMENT

Inconsistent sexual response

When the sexual dysfunction either continues uninterrupted, or reoccurs periodically, the therapist should suspect that certain residual elements of the original precipitating problems have not been dealt with adequately; or it may be that new conflicts have arisen, and they are now inhibiting the afflicted sexual response cycle. In either case, extended care -- often individual and/or conjoint psychotherapy -- will be necessary.

In particular circumstances, such as with reoccurring premature ejaculation, the couple may simply need to be told that they should continue to practice the "squeeze" or "start-stop" treatments on their own. Often this "self treatment" will be sufficient to control the dysfunctional symptoms. Sometimes, however, the couple will not apply themselves, or resistance will set in, and on-going supervision by the sex therapist will be necessary.

Patient dissatisfaction

Occasionally, one or both partners will not be satisfied with the degree of progress that has been made. That is to say, a formerly preorgastic woman may now be dissatisfied because she cannot climax via coitus even though she is easily responsive through either masturbation or oral sex; or it may be that a diabetic male may be disappointed in the firmness of his erectile response. When problems of this type occur, extended care may be warranted.

Obviously, not every sexual disorder can be corrected, and not everyone can learn to be responsive under all circumstances. When these limitations are evident, however, or when the patient (or the couple) maintains unrealistic expectations, on-going sex education, psychotherapy, and/or relationship counseling may help them to understand their situation more realistically.

Continued treatment

Ideally, of course, sex therapy will consist of intensive treatments that have been undertaken for a brief period. Unfortunately, not everyone is able to resolve their conflicts quickly; this means that extended treatment will sometimes be necessary, and it is the realistic sex therapist that provides for this possibility.

FOLLOW-UP TREATMENT

After the patients have discontinued regular contact with the sex therapist, follow-up evaluations may be valuable indicators of the lasting effects of treatment. These "check-ups" should be undertaken at least twice; the first should occur between thirty and sixty days after treatment has concluded, the second should be undertaken at the end of the first year. (Because economic factors may prevent certain patients from returning, these evaluations should be at no charge; in this way patient participation will not be discouraged.)

Short-term follow-up

Patients are probably most vulnerable to recurring sexual inhibition during the first sixty days after treatment. This is most certainly due to a variety of factors but the most obvious reason is that it is relatively easy for persons to return to old habits (e.g., drinking, smoking, premature ejaculation, etc.), even when those habits are painful and/or destructive. Therefore, an early check-up, during the first sixty days of the recovery period, may help to identify a relapse -- or potential relapse -- situation, and quick intervention should be able to prevent a firm reconditioning of the sexual inhibition.

There is no particular pattern, or diagnostic format, that is regularly used for this evaluation.[1] Most often, however, a conjoint office consultation will be sufficient to explore the post-treatment situation. During this session the therapist can also make constructive recommendations about particular problems, or suggest that the patients return to treatment, if necessary.

Long-term follow-up

If the sexual dysfunction has not returned, nor another developed, by the end of the first twelve-month period, it may be that treatment has been successful. On the other hand, anyone, at any time, is vulnerable to sexual inhibitions, therefore, on-going vigilance is necessary in all cases.

---

[1]Follow-up procedures and techniques have been sorely neglected in the sex therapy literature. For instance, not one major text or professional journal devotes specific attention to this important area of patient care.

Notes:

This twelve-month follow-up is simply a precautionary measure that will make it possible for the patients to focus their attentions on their sexual relationships, while obtaining the informed opinion of a neutral third party. Here, also, problems can be noted and recommendations made: occasionally some patients may even need to be returned to treatment at this point. Naturally, follow-up does not have to stop at this point; ongoing consultations may continue at whatever intervals patients and therapists negotiate.

In addition to being helpful to patients, these evaluations should also be instructive to therapists who may be able to get some impression of their clinical effectiveness by noting the return or absence of the sexual disorders over a long period. Naturally, other contributing factors, both positive and negative, must also be taken into account, but similar results, recurring over a reasonable period of time, may have some validity as a comment on the quality of patient care the therapist is providing.

BIBLIOGRAPHY

Allison, J., and Wilson, W. Sexual behavior in
manic patients. Southern Journal of Medicine,
1960, 53. 870-874.

American Medical Association Committee on Human
Sexuality. Human Sexuality. Chicago, 1972.

Annon, J.S. The Behavioral Treatment of Sexual
problems: Intensive Therapy. Honolulu: Enabling Systems, Inc., 1975a.

Annon, J.S. The Sexual Fear Inventory--Male
Form. Honolulu: Enabling Systems, Inc.,
1975b.

Annon, J.S. The Sexual Fear Inventory--Male
Form. Honolulu: Enabling Systems, Inc.,
1975c.

Aquinas, T. Summa Theologica (Vols. 1-3).
(The Fathers of the English Dominican Province,
trans.) New York: Bonziger Bros., 1947.

Barbach, L.G. For Yourself: The Fulfillment of
Female Sexuality. New York: Signet Books
1975.

Blakeney, P., Kinder, B., Creson, D., Powell, L.,
and Sutton, C. A short-term intensive workshop approach for the treatment of human sexual inadequacy. Journal of Sex and Marital
Therapy, 1976, 2, 124-129.

Boyarsky, R.E., and Boyarsky, S. Urological and
behavioral approach to the treatment of secondary impotence. The Journal of Urology, 1978,
119, 229-230.

Cassidy, W., Flanagan, N., Spellman, M., and Cohne,
M. Clinical observations in manic depressive
disease. Journal of the American Medical Association, 1957, 164, 1535-1546.

Chilgren, R.A. and Briggs, M.M. On being explicit.
Siecus Report, May 1973, p.1.

Colgan, A. Female sexual dysfunction. New Zeal-
and Nursing Forum, 1977, 5 (1), 8-11.

Ellis, A. An informal history of sex therapy.
The Counseling Psychologist, 1975, 5 (1),
9-13.

Ellison, C. Psychosomatic factors in the uncon-
summated marriage. Journal of Psychomatic
Research, 1968, 12, 61.

Ellison, C. Vaginismus. Medical Aspects of Human Sexuality, 1972, 6 (8), 34.

Eysenck, H. Personality and sexual adjustment.
British Journal of Psychiatry, 1971, 118,
593-608.

Farkas, G.M., and Rosen, R.C. Effect of alcohol
on elicited male sexual responses. Journal
of Studies on Alcohol, 1976, 37, 265-272.

Notes:

Fay, A. Sexual problems related to poor communication. Medical Aspects of Human Sexuality, 1977, 11 (16), 48-52; 55; 59; 60.

Fenichel, O. The Psychoanalytic Theory of Neurosis. New York: W.W. Norton, 1945.

Fertel, N. Vaginismus: a review. Journal of Sex and Marital Therapy. 1977, 3, 113-121.

Fisher, S. and Osofsky, H. Sexual responsiveness in women. Archives of General Psychiatry, 1967, 17, 214-226.

Fogarty, T.F. Sexual estrangement in marriage. Medical Aspects of Human Sexuality, 1977, 11 (4), 122-123; 127-129; 133; 135.

Franks, C.M. and Wilson, G.T. Behavior therapy and sexual disorders: commentary. In C.M. Franks and G.T. Wilson (Eds.), Annual Review of Behavior Therapy. New York: Brunner/Mazel, 1974.

Freedman, M. Sexual behavior of American college women; an empirical study and a historical survey. Merrill-Palmer, 1965, 11, 33-48.

Freud, S. Collected Papers (Vol. 5). New York: Basic Books, 1959.

Fuchs, K. Hoch, Z., and Abramovici, H. Vaginismus: the hypno-therapeutic approach. Journal of Sex Research, 1975, 11, 39.

Fuchs, K. Hoch, Z., and Paldo, E. Hypno-desensitization therapy of vaginismus. International Journal of Clinical Experimental Hypnosis, 1973, 21, 144.

Furlow, W.L. Surgical management of impotence using the inflatable penile prosthesis. Mayo Clinic Proceedings, 1976, 51, 325-328.

Geboes, K., Omer, S., and DeMoor, P. Primary anejaculation: diagnosis and therapy. Fertility and Sterility, 1975, 26, 1018-1020.

Goldberg, M. Selective impotence. Medical Aspects of Human Sexuality, 1972, b, 90-102.

Graber, B., and Kline-Graber, G. How a woman can assist an impotent man. Medical Aspects of Human Sexuality, 1977, 11 (4), 58-67.

Fuchs, K. Hoch, Z., and Abramovici, H. Vaginismus: the hypno-therapeutic approach. Journal of Sex Research, 1975, 11, 39.

Fuchs, K. Hoch, Z., and Paldo, E. Hypno-desensitization therapy of vaginismus. International Journal of Clinical Experimental Hypnosis, 1973, 21, 144.

Furlow, W.L. Surgical management of impotence using the inflatable penile prosthesis. Mayo Clinic Proceedings, 1976, 51, 325-328.

Geboes, K., Omer, S., and DeMoor, P. Primary anejaculation: diagnosis and therapy. Fertility and Sterility, 1975, 26, 1018-1020.

Goldberg, M. Selective impotence. Medical Aspects of Human Sexuality, 1972, b, 90-102.

Graber, B., and Kline-Graber, G. How a woman

can assist an impotent man. Medical Aspects of Human Sexuality, 1977, 11 (4), 58-67.

Hartman, W.E. and Fithian, M.A. Treatment of sexual dysfunction: a bio-psycho-social approach. Long Beach: Center for Marital and Sexual Studies, 1972.

Huffman, J. Office gynecology: some facts about the clitoris. Postgraduate Medicine, 1976, 60 (5), 245-247.

Hunt, M. "Sexual behavior in the 1970's." Playboy, 1973, 20 (10), pp. 84-88; 194-207.

Isenberg, S., and Elting, L. "A guide to sexual surgery." Cosmopolitan, November 1976, pp. 104; 108; 110, 164-165.

Jankovich, R. and Miller, P. Response of women with primary orgasmic dysfunction to audiovisual education. Journal of Sex and Marital Therapy, 1978, 4, 16-19.

Jeffcoate, T.N.A. cited by Kinch, R.A.H. Painful coitus. Medical Aspects of Human Sexuality, 1967, 1, 8.

Johnson, D. Marriage Counseling: Theory and Practice. New York: Prentice-Hall, 1961.

Kales, J.D., Martin, E.D.., and Franchini, D. Treating sexual dysfunctions in male patients. Pennsylvania Medicine, Dec. 1977, pp. 38-43.

Kaplan, H.S. The classification of the female sexual dysfunctions. Journal of Sex and Marital Therapy, 1974a, 1, 124-138.

Kaplan, H.S. The New Sex Therapy: Active Treatment of Sexual Dysfunction. New York: Brunner/Mazel, 1974b.

Kaplan, H.S. The Illustrated Manual of Sex Therapy. New York: Quadrangle, 1975.

Kaplan, H.S. Editorial: towards a rational classification of the sexual dysfunctions. Journal of Sex and Marital Therapy, 1976, 2, 83; 84/

Kaplan, H.S. Hypoactive sexual desire. Journal of Sex and Marital Therapy, 1977, 3, 3-9.

Kaplan, H.S. Disorders of Sexual Desire and Other New Concepts and Techniques in Sex Therapy. New York: Simon and Schuster, 1979.

Kaplan, H.S., Kohl, R.N., Pomeroy, W.B., Offit, A.K., and Hogan, B. Group treatment of premature ejaculation. Archives of Sexual Behavior, 1974, 3, 443-452.

Kelly, G.L. Sex Manual for Those Married or About To Be. Augusta, Ga.: Southern Medical Supply Company, 1953.

Kelly, G.L. Sexual Feeling in Women. Augusta, Ga.: Elkay, 1930.

Kent, S. Impotence as a consequence of organic disease. Geriatrics, Sept. 1975, p.p. 155; 157.

Kinsey, A.C. Sex behavior in the human animal. Annual New York Academy of Science, 1947, 47, 635-637.

Kinsey, A.C., Sexual Behavior in the Human Female. Philadelphia: W.B. Saunders, 1953.

Notes:

Kinsey, A.C., Pomeroy, W.B., and Martin, C.E. Sexual Behavior in the Human Male. Philadelphia: W.B. Saunders, 1948.

Kirker, W., and Kirker, J. The sexological procedure. Unpublished paper, 1980.

Kleegman, S. Frigidity in women. Quarterly Review of Surgery in Obstetrics and Gynecology. 1959, 16, 243-245.

Kohlenberg, R. Directed masturbation and the treatment of primary orgasmic dysfunction. Archives of Sexual Behavior, 1974, 3, 349-356.

Krohne, E.C. Code words: aids to articulation in sex therapy. Paper presented at the A.A.S.E. C.T. Second Annual Southeastern Regional Conference, Asheville, N.C., 1977.

Landis, C., Bollis, M., and D'Esopo, D. Psychological and physical concomitants of adjustment in marriage. Human Biology, 1940, 12, 559-565.

Lazarus, A. The treatment of chronic frigidity by systematic desensitization. Journal of Nervous and Mental Disorders, 1963, 136, 276-278.

Lazarus, A. Modes of treatment for sexual inadequacies. Medical Aspects of Human Sexuality, 1969, 3, 53.

Levine, S.B. Marital sexual dysfunction: ejaculation disturbances. Annals of Internal Medicine, 1976a, 84, 575-579.

Levine, S.B. Marital sexual dysfunction: erectile dysfunction. Annals of Internal Medicine, 1976b, 85, 342-350.

Levine S.B. Some thoughts about the pathogenesis of premature ejaculation. Journal of Sex and Marital Therapy, 1975, 1, 326-334.

Levine, S.B., and Agle, D. The effectiveness of sex therapy for chronic secondary psychological impotence. Journal of Sex and Marital Therapy, 1978, 4, 235-258.

Light and Life. Charlotte, N.C.: C.H. Robinson and Co., no date.

Lobitz, W.C., and LoPiccolo, J. Clinical innovations in the behavioral treatment of sexual dysfunction. In A.S. Gurman and D.C. Rice (Eds.) Couples in Conflict. New York: Jason Aronson, 1975.

LoPiccolo, J., and Lobitz, W. The role of masturbation in the treatment of orgasmic dysfunction. Archives of Sexual Behavior, 1972, 2, 163-171.

Lording, D.W. Impotence: role of drug and hormonal treatment, Drugs, 1978, 15 (2) 144-150.

Mann, J., and Katsuranis, J. The dynamics and problems of sexual relationships. Postgraduate Medicine, 1975, 58 (1), 79-86.

Masters, W.H. and Johnson, V.E. Human sexual response, Boston: Little, Brown & Co., 1966.

Masters, W.H. and Johnson, V.E. Human Sexual In-
    adequacy. Boston: Little, Brown & Co., 1970.
Meyer, J.K. Sexual problems in office practice:
    guidelines for identification and management.
    In J.K. Meyer (Ed.), Clinical Management of
    Sexual Disorders. Baltimore: Williams and
    Wilkins, 1976.
Miller, H., and Wilson, W. Relation of sexual be-
    haviors, values and conflicts to avowed hap-
    piness and personal adjustments. Psychologi-
    cal Report, 1968, 23, 1075-1860.
Munjack, D., and Staples, F. Psychological chara-
    cteristics of women with sexual inhibition
    (frigidity) in sex clinics. Journal of Nervous
    and Mental Diseases, 1976, 163, 117-123.
Noonan, J.T., Jr., Contraception. Cambridge:
    Belknap Press, 1966.
O'Connor, J.F. Effectiveness of psychological
    treatment of human sexual dysfunction. Clini-
    cal Obstretics and Gynecology, 1976, 19, 449-
    464.
O'Connor, J.F. and Stern, L.O. The results of
    treatment in functional sexual disorders, New
    York State Journal of Medicine, August, 1972,
    1927-1934.
Osborne, D. Psychologic evaluation of impotent
    men. Mayo Clinic Proceedings, 1976, 51, 363-
    366.
Paine, W. A Treatise on the Principles and Prac-
    tices of Medicine and Pathology, Diseases of
    Women and Children, and Surgery, Philadelphia,
    Pub. Soc., 1866.
Pion, R.J. The Sexual Response Profile. Honolulu:
    Enabling Systems, Inc., 1975.
Popoff, L.M. A simple method for the diagnosis
    of depression by the family physician. Clini-
    cal Medicine, 1969a, 76, 24-29.
Popoff, L.M. The Index of Depression, Ardsley,
    New York: 1969b.
Purtell, J., Robins, E., and Cohn, M. Observations
    of clinical aspects of hysteria. Journal of
    the American Medical Association, 1951, 146,
    902-909.
Racy, J. How sexual relationships mirror the total
    relationship. Medical Aspects of Human Sex-
    uality, 1977, 11 (8), 98; 103; 107; 109; 113-114.
Reed, D.M. Eight reasons for failure in sex thera-
    py. Medical Aspects of Human Sexuality, 1976,
    10 (5), 134-139.
Reich, W. The Function of the Orgasm. (V.R. Car-
    fagno, trans). New York: Pocket Books, 1975.
Renshaw, D.C. Doxepin treatment of sexual dys-
    functions associated with depression. In J.
    Mendels (Ed.), Excerpta Medica, Princeton,
    N.J.: American Elsevier Pub. Co., Inc. 1975.
Renshaw, D.C. Sexual dysfunctions. In A. Kiev
    (Ed.), Somatic Manifestations of Depressive

Notes:

Notes:

Disorders. London: Excerpta Medica, 1974.

Renshaw, D.C. Impotence--some causes and cures. _American Family Practitioner_, 1978, 17 (2), 143-146.

Robie, W.F. _The Art of Love_. Ithaca, N.Y.: Rational Life Press, 1925.

Robie, W.F. _Rational Sex Ethics_. Ithaca, N.Y.: Rational Life Press, 1927.

Robinson, C.H., and Annon. J.S. _The Heterosexual Attitude Scale--Female Form_. Honolulu: Enabling Systems, Inc., 1975a.

Robinson, C.H. and Annon, J.S. _The Heterosexual Attitude Scale--Male Form_. Honolulu: Enabling Systems, Inc., 1975b.

ROCOM Health History Questionnaire, Patient Care Systems, 1972.

Rubin, I. Sexual adjustments in relation to pregnancy, illness, surgery, physical handicaps and other unusual circumstances. In C.E. Vincent (Ed.), _Human Sexuality in Medical Education and Practice_. Springfield, Ill.: Charles C. Thomas, 1968.

Sager, C.J. A false dichotomy. _Journal of Sex and Marital Therapy_, 1975, 1, 187-189.

Schneidman, B. and McGuire L. Group therapy for nonorgasmic women: two age levels. _Archives of Sex Therapy_. 1956, 5, 239-247.

Seagraves, R.T. Primary orgasmic dysfunction: essential treatment components. _Journal of Sex and Marital Therapy_, 1976, 2, 115-123.

Semans, J.H. Premature ejaculation: a new approach. _Southern Medical Journal_, 1956, 49, 353-357.

Serafetinides, E.A. Assessing the sexual side effects of psychotropic drugs. _Hospital Physician_, Jan. 1972, pp. 58-60.

Sethney, H.T., and Roy, J.B. Impotence--management with penile prosthesis. _Journal of the Oklahoma State Medical Association_, 1976. 69, 428.

Shiller, P. _Creative Approach to Sex Education and Counseling_. New York: Association Press, 1973.

Snyder, A., LoPiccolo, L., and LoPiccolo, J. Secondary orgasmic dysfunction II. Case study. _Archives of Sexual Behavior_. 1975, 4, 227-283.

Sotile, W., Kilmann, P., Fellingstad, D. A sexual enhancement workshop: beyond group systematic desensitization for women's sexual anxiety. _Journal of Sex and Marital Therapy_, 1977, 3, 249-255.

Spano, L. and Lamont, J. Dyspareunia, a symptom of female sexual dysfunction. _The Canadian Nurse_, August, 1975, pp. 22-25

Taylor, R.W. Aspects of sexual medicine: some of the commoner sexual dysfunctions--problems mainly affecting males. _The British Medical_

Journal, 1975, 2, 739-741.

Terman, L. *Psychological factors in marital happiness*. New York: McGraw-Hill, 1938.

Uddenberg, N. Psychological aspects of sexual inadequacy in women. *Journal of Psychosomatic Research*, 1974, 18, 33-47.

Wabrek, A.J., and Wabrek, C.J. Premature ejaculation. Connecticut Medicine, 1977, 41, 214-216.

Wahl, C.W. Psychiatric techniques in the taking of a sexual history. In C.W. Wahl (Ed.), *Sexual Problems, Diagnosis and Treatment in Medical Practice*. New York: The Free Press, 1967.

Winokur, G. Sexual behavior: its relationship to certain affects and psychiatric diseases. In G. Winokur (Ed.), *Determinants of Human Sexual Behavior*. Springfield, Ill.: Charles C. Thomas, 1963.

Winokur, G., and Gaston, W. Sex, anger and anxiety: intrapersonal interaction in married couples. *Diseases of the Nervous System, 1961*. 22, 256-260.

Winokur, G. and Holeman, E. Chronic anxiety neurosis: clinical and sexual aspects. *Aeta Psychiatry*, 1963, 39, 384-412.

Wolpe, J. *Psychotherapy by Reciprocal Inhibition*. Stanford: Stanford University Press, 1958.

Wolpe, J. *The Practice of Behavior Therapy*. New York: Pergamon, 1969.

Zung, W.W.K. A self-rating depression scale. *Archives of General Psychiatry*, 1965 12, 63.

Zung, W.W.K. Depression in the normal aged. *Psychosomatics*, 8, Sept.-Oct. 1967a.

Zung, W.W.K. Factors influencing the self-rating depression scale. *Archives of General Psychiatry*, 1967, 16, 543b.

Zung, W.W.K. *The Measurement of Depression: a Self Rating Depression Scale*. Lakeside Laboratories, Milwaukee, rev. ed. 1967c.

Zung, W.W.K. Richards, C.B., and Short, M.J. Self-rating depression scale in an outpatient clinic. *Archives of General Psychiatry*, 1965 13, 508.

Zussman, L., and Zussman, S. Continuous time-limited treatment of standard sexual disorders. In J.K. Meyer (Ed.), *Clinical Management of Sexual Disorders*. Baltimore: Williams and Wilkins, 1976.

Notes:

INDEX